Andréa Maria Góes Negrão

Bubalinos as Renal Carriers of Leptospira sp in Marajó - Amazonia

Andréa Maria Góes Negrão

Bubalinos as Renal Carriers of Leptospira sp in Marajó - Amazonia

Serologic prevalence and renal carrier status in Marajoa buffaloes from the Arari micro-region, Pará, Brazil

ScienciaScripts

Imprint
Any brand names and product names mentioned in this book are subject to trademark, brand or patent protection and are trademarks or registered trademarks of their respective holders. The use of brand names, product names, common names, trade names, product descriptions etc. even without a particular marking in this work is in no way to be construed to mean that such names may be regarded as unrestricted in respect of trademark and brand protection legislation and could thus be used by anyone.

Cover image: www.ingimage.com

This book is a translation from the original published under ISBN 978-613-9-62349-5.

Publisher:
Sciencia Scripts
is a trademark of
Dodo Books Indian Ocean Ltd. and OmniScriptum S.R.L publishing group

120 High Road, East Finchley, London, N2 9ED, United Kingdom
Str. Armeneasca 28/1, office 1, Chisinau MD-2012, Republic of Moldova, Europe
Printed at: see last page
ISBN: 978-620-7-72175-7

SUMMARY

DEDICATORY

I dedicate this book to my son Lucas, may he

may all his dreams come true.

SUMMARY

The presence of *Leptospira spp* was verified using direct and indirect laboratory diagnostic techniques in buffaloes belonging to 10 herds in the Arari micro-region, Marajó Archipelago, State of Parà, Amazon Region, Brazil. The indirect demonstration techniques (serological tests) used were Microscopic Serum Agglutination (SAM) and Rapid Macroagglutination (MAR), and Isolation in culture medium and Polymerase Chain Reaction (PCR), as techniques for direct demonstration of the agent. A total of 53% of animals were found to be positive by SAM and the most prevalent serovars were Butembo (49.05%), Hardjo (40.57%), Autumnalis (3.77%), Pomona and Castellonis (1.87% each) and Bratislava, Pyrogenes and Shermani (0.95% each). By MAR, the prevalence found was 27.5% positive, with 19.5% of the animals proving positive to both tests. All the herds were prevalent in both tests, ranging from 30 to 75% by SAM and 15 to 50% by MAR. *Leptospira spp.* was found in 13 buffalo by culture isolation. Of these, ten animals showed the agent only in the kidney, two animals showed it in the kidney and urine, and one animal showed it only in the urine. The serovars that reacted in the animals that tested positive for kidney isolation were: Butembo (six samples), Hardjo (five samples) and Autumnalis (one sample). In the urine samples, only the Hardjo serovar was reactive. PCR did not show the bacteria in any kidney or urine sample. It can be concluded that leptospirosis is widespread in the Marajoa buffalo herds studied, including the presence of *Leptospira spp* in kidney and/or urine samples. Key words: Leptospira, bubalinos, prevalence, isolation, Marajó.

1. INTRODUCTION

1.1 Disease definition

Ieptospirosis is a zoonotic infectious disease that occurs in many species of domestic and wild animals, and accidentally affects humans. It has a cosmopolitan distribution and is considered endemic in Brazil and particularly in the Amazon (Vasconcellos *et al.,* 1997; Negrao *et al.,* 2003).

The disease affects domestic food-producing animals such as cattle, buffalo, pigs and goats, and causes high economic losses due to abortions, births of weak animals that may or may not survive, infertility, increased calving intervals, agalactia with reduced milk production and risks of human contamination (Ellis, 1994). There is also data on mortality in affected herds (Cascelli *et al.,* 1979). It is known that when there is a drop in milk production and abortions, the infection has been present on the farm for at least seven years. The financial consequences are abortion rates of 1 to 18%, a reduction in milk production of up to 50% of cows and a drop in production of 10 to 30% per year (Genovez, 1999).

The impact of leptospirosis on the production and productivity indices of buffalo herds needs to be clarified, as does the identification of serological variants that occur in the region, thus facilitating preventive and/or therapeutic measures. To this end, it is necessary to prove the presence of leptospires in blood serum, urine and kidney samples from buffaloes destined for slaughter.

1.2 General considerations about buffaloes

Buffalo are domestic animals of the bovid family, classified in the sub-family Bovinae, genus *Bubalis,* divided into two main groups: *Bubalus bubalis,* also known as river buffalo, and *Bubalus bubalis var. kerebau,* known as swamp buffalo (ABCB, 2005).

The buffalo species is seen as a very good farming option, with great adaptability, wide use in animal traction and excellent meat and milk production (Cockrill, 1994). Bubalinos have a docile temperament, which makes them easy to breed and manage, and they adapt well to a wide variety of environmental conditions. They can produce meat in less time and more economically than cattle (Oliveira *et al.,* 2005).

The use of buffalo as traction animals in the Amazon region is traditional, especially in flooded areas. They are used to transport goods and pull canoes when river water levels are low. They are also used to transport wood and to plow land on small properties (Martinez, 2002).

In Brazil, the production chain for buffalo meat is still disorganized, due to the scarcity of studies involving the production and technology of buffalo meat. In slaughterhouses, there is a clear interruption in the production chain, and the most common occurrence is the mixing of buffalo meat with beef, as they are similar in taste and appearance (Gangleazzi, *et al.*, 2003).

According to the Brazilian Association of Buffalo Breeders, four breeds are recognized in Brazil: Mediterranean, Murrah, Jafarabadi and Carabao. The Mediterràneo breed is of Italian origin and is suitable for both meat and milk production. The Murrah breed, of Indian origin, presents animals with medium and compact conformation, light heads and short, spiral horns. The Jafarabadi, also from India, is the largest breed, with long, thin horns and a long curvature. The Carabao breed is the only one adapted to swampy regions and is concentrated on the island of Marajó. It originated in the north of the Philippines and has a lighter coat, a triangular head, large, pointed horns, medium size and the ability to produce meat and milk, as well as being widely used as a driving force (ABCB, 2005).

According to data from IBGE's 2005 Municipal Livestock Survey (IBGE, 2005), Brazil's cattle and buffalo herds total 207,156,696 and 1,173,629 head, respectively. In the state of Parà, these herds number 18,063,669 cattle and 466,210 buffalo.

The Marajó Archipelago, located at the mouth of the Amazon River in the state of Parà, has a geographical area of approximately 49,600 km^2 and is made up of a group of islands that constitute the largest river island in the world. The Marajó mesoregion is a subdivision of the state, created by the IBGE, which brings together 16 municipalities with similar economic and social characteristics. This mesoregion is the Brazilian region with the highest concentration of buffaloes, with 308,826 head, but the cattle population is higher, with 349,114 head. This mesoregion, seen in Figure 1, is divided into three micro-regions: Arari, Furos de Breves and Portel (IBGE, 2005).

The Arari micro-region covers an area of 28,948.830 kms and has the largest herds, with 321,162 head of cattle and 290,168 head of buffalo, respectively. It is divided into seven municipalities with the following buffalo herds: Cachoeira do Arari (35,800 head), Chaves (150,000), Muanà (14,400), Ponta de Pedras (20,000), Salvaterra (15,700), Santa Cruz do Arari (23,000) and Soure (31,000). The Furos de Breves micro-region covers an area of 30,094.393 km^2 and has a cattle herd of 7,867 head and a buffalo herd of 12,205 head. It is divided into five municipalities: Afuà, Anajàs, Breves, Curralinho and Sao Sebastiao da Boa Vista. The Portel micro-region is divided into four municipalities: Bagre, Gurupà, Melgaço and Portel, and has an area of 45,096.076 km2. The number of cattle and buffalo in the Portel micro-region is 20,085 and 6,453, respectively (IBGE, 2005; ADEPARA, 2007).

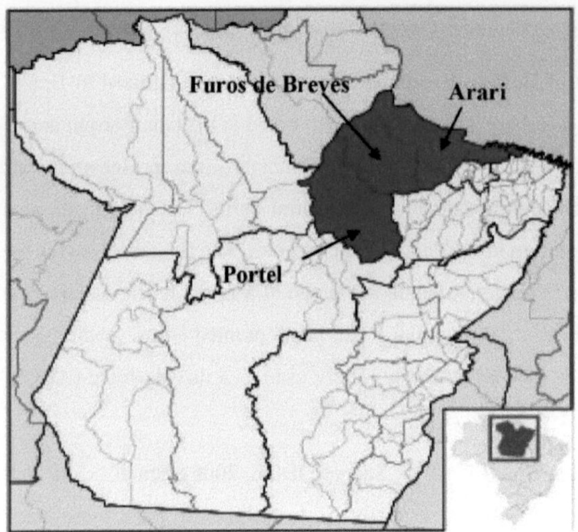

Figure 1 - Illustrative map of the mesoregions of the state of Parà, highlighting the Marajó mesoregion and its three micro-regions (IBGE, 2005; Wikipedia, 2006).

1.3 Etiology

Leptospirosis is caused by bacteria of the genus *Leptospira,* which are obligate aerobes, spiral-shaped, flexible and mobile, and measure from 6 to 20 μm in length and 0.1 μm in diameter. They grow best at a temperature of 28 to 30° C and a pH of 7.2 to 7.6, and are very sensitive to deviations from these values. They are also highly sensitive to common phenol-based disinfectants and those with a pH below six and above eleven (Veronesi, 1991).

The genus *Leptospira* was initially divided into two species: *Leptospira interrogans* and *Leptospira biflexa.* Based on serological criteria, serogroups and serovars of pathogenic and saprophytic leptospires were included. Today, through DNA sequencing, there is a new division for this genus into ten species (Table 1), with the pathogenic leptospires being divided into three groups as shown below: group 1 with *Leptospira interrogans* and Leptospira *kirschneri*; group 2 with Leptospira *borgpetersenii, Leptospira weilli* and Leptospira *santarosai and* group 3 with Leptospira *nogucchii* and Leptospira *meyeri*. The intermediate leptospira is Leptospira *inadai* and the saprophytic species are *Leptospira biflexa* and *Leptospira woibacchu* (Ellis, 1995).

Leptospires are made up of 26 serogroups, which are made up of serovars, and thus determined according to cross-antigenic characteristics (Ellis, 1995). The serogroups have the practical purpose of grouping together strains of serovars that have antigenic similarities. This grouping is necessary in view of the large number of leptospiral serovars already classified (Korver, 2000).

Serovars are the taxonomic units of leptospires and are characterized by their agglutination absorption patterns (Jawetz *et al.,* 1991). Two hundred and fifty-five (255) serovars in the Leptospiraceae family have already been found (Ellis, 1995). The definition of serovar was not only for systematic purposes, but also for practical application and description of primary and secondary host relationships (Yasuda *et al.,* 1987; Korver, 2000).

Table 1 - Classification of *Leptospira spp* species (Ellis, 1995).

Order Spirochaetales	
Family Leptospiraceae	
Genres	Species
Turneria	*Turneria parva* (formerly *Leptospira parva*)
Leptonema	*Leptospira illini*
Group 1	*Leptospira interrogans* and *Leptospira kirschineri*
Pathogenic Group 2	*Leptospira borgpetersenii, L. weilli* and *L. Santarosai*
Leptospira	
Group 3	*Leptospira nogucchii* and *L.meyeri*
Intermediate	*Leptospira inadai*
Saprophytes	*Leptospira biflexa* and *L. woibacchu*

1.4 Epidemiology

All animal species are sensitive to leptospires, but in production animals, pigs and cattle are the most sensitive, with marked differences depending on the serovar and its virulence (Ellis & McDowell, 1993). Buffaloes are also sensitive to different serovars of leptospires (Chaudhry *et al.*, 1996).

Bovine leptospirosis is distributed worldwide, occurring at any age and in both sexes. Infection is favored in tropical and subtropical regions due to the survival of leptospira for long periods in humid environments, thus contaminating susceptible animals with infected urine and increasing the opportunity for exposure (Ellis, 1984). The risk factors on the farm are: water, wet pasture, contaminated and shared breeding stock and the purchase of animals without prior quarantine or serological analysis (Genovez, 1999).

Many animal species serve as hosts for leptospira, and each serovar has one or more of these hosts, which are better adapted to them, just as the hosts or reservoirs are better adapted to one or more of these serovars (Kopcha & Bartlett, 1997).

There are occasions when the prevalence of leptospirosis can increase because some animals become carriers for some time or intermittently. Although a small number of serovars are endemic in a given region or country, an animal species will be infected by serovars maintained by one or more species present in that region (Ellis & McDowell, 1993).

According to Ellis (1984), bovine leptospirosis is transmitted in two situations, the first being when strains are adapted and transmitted by cattle, as in the case of the Hardjo serovar, in which there is transmission from cattle to cattle, and is independent of region and rainfall. In the second case, transmission occurs when strains are maintained by other species which are present in the region and which, through direct or indirect contact, cause accidental infections in cattle and buffalo. The prevalence of accidental infections also depends on the survival of the leptospira outside the host.

The most important serovars causing infections in cattle are Hardjo, which they maintain. Accidental infections are caused by the serovars Pomona, Grippotyphosa, Icterohaemorrhagiae, Canicola and Bratislava (Ellis & McDowell, 1993). Ciceroni *et al.* (1995) tried to demonstrate that the buffalo species could also act as a host for Hardjo by attempting to isolate it from urine samples and serologically testing 436 blood serum samples. Although they found 67% of total positive samples by serology, no leptospira strain was isolated.

Animal leptospirosis is transmitted through the main source of contamination, which is contaminated urine, but other excreta are also important, such as uterine discharge, placenta and semen, which are sources of direct and indirect contamination from one animal to another (sick and/or carriers). By eliminating large quantities of leptospires with their urine, they contaminate pastures, stables and the water of lakes and rivers, creating sources of contamination for humans and animals (Bolin *et al.,* 1991; Ellis, 1994).

Urinary excretion depends on the adaptation of the serovar to the host. When infection occurs in a host that maintains the serovar, there is infection in the organs for a long time, and perhaps for life; however, in the case of infection in an accidental host, colonization is short-lived and urinary excretion may not occur (Ellis & McDowell, 1993).

Cattle show leptospirosis for a period of between 10 and 118 days, on average 36 days. However, it can reach longer periods of up to 180 days after the onset of infection (Beer, 1988). According to Leonard *et al.* (1992), leptospirosis in cattle infected experimentally via the intrauterine route lasts an average of 182 days and via the conjunctival route 224 days, with no evidence of seasonal excretion.

In the case of Hardj o infections in cattle, the intensity of excretion is greater during the first four to six weeks of elimination, with leptospirosis being more constant during this period. However, when venereal infections occur, such as the Bratislava serovar in pigs, urinary excretion is of low intensity (Ellis & McDowell, 1993).

Bielanski *et al.* (1998) experimentally infected 30 herds with *Leptospira* Hardjo via the cervical, conjunctival, intranasal and uterine routes and managed to establish infection in the reproductive tract in all the herds, but ruled out the possibility of transmission via embryo transfer. However, Heinemann *et al.* (2000) detected the Andamana, Brasiliensis, Buenos Aires, Butembo, Garcia, Rufino and Whitcombi serovars by PCR in experimentally infected bovine semen samples from artificial insemination centers in Brazil, proving the importance of venereal transmission of bovine leptospirosis through artificial insemination.

The occurrence of leptospirosis with serology or the isolation of the bacteria have been reported in buffaloes in Thailand, India, Pakistan, China, the Philippines, Bulgaria and Egypt (Khan & Khan, 1988). In Pakistan, Ahmed (1990) isolated leptospires from the milk of buffaloes that had mastitis with flaccid udders.

In Brazil, the first serological surveys of buffalo were carried out in Sao Paulo in the 1970s and 1980s, and showed percentages of positive animals of 6.85%, 6.72%, 16.6%, 22.4% and 30.77%, with a predominance of the Wolffi, Pomona, Grippotyphosa and Icterohaemorrhagiae serovars. However, the antigen collections used were very different and the cut-off point set for serum screening also varied (Santa Rosa *et al.,* 1970; Sandoval *et al.,* 1979; Giorgi *et al.,* 1981; Yasuda et al, 1982; Girio, 1984). In Bahia, Dória *et al.* (1979) found 59.70% of seroreactive buffaloes, with a predominance of the Wolffi serovar.

Langoni *et al.* (1997) found 152 seropositive buffaloes out of 403 examined (37.7%) in the Vale da Ribeira, SP. Also in Sao Paulo, seropositivity in buffalo was found in 43.7% of the animals, with a predominance of the Hardjo and Wolffi serovars (Fâvero *et al.,* 2002).

In cattle, other serological findings were shown by Vasconcellos *et al.* (1997) who examined 2449 cattle from 56 properties in six Brazilian states (Minas Gerais, Sao Paulo, Rio de Janeiro, Mato Grosso do Sul, Paranà, Rio Grande do Sul) and found 60.4% seropositive with a prevalence of Hardjo, Wolffi, Pomona, Grippotyphosa and Australis. Oliveira *et al.* (2001) analyzed 464 cattle from 15 herds in the state of Pernambuco and found 47.63% of positive samples, with a predominance of Hardjo, Bratislava, Castellonis and Tarassovi.

It is important to mention that Moreira (1994) isolated the Hardjo and Georgia serovars from the urine of cows with reproductive problems for the first time in Brazil. However, Langoni *et al* (1999) investigated the presence of leptospires in the kidneys of 120 aborted fetuses, and analyzed maternal paired serology (on the day of abortion and 15 days after). Isolation was positive in 15 samples, four for Hardjo, three for Pomona and eight for Wolffi.

In the buffalo species, Vasconcellos *et al.* (2001) isolated *Leptospira santarosai*, serovar Guaricura from buffalo urine samples. Several serovars have been isolated from biological samples of domestic animals, as shown in Table 2.

In the state of Parà, little research has been done on leptospirosis in humans and domestic animals, most of which has been carried out on bovine and bubaline species. Lins *et al.* (1986) evaluated the occurrence of anti-leptospiral agglutinins in 54 cattle, finding 9.3% (five animals) positive, where four animals reacted to Wolffi and one to Australis. Moreira (1982) analyzed animals from Parà and Amazonas using MAR. In Parà, of the 1,487 serological samples analyzed, Hardjo was found in 21.7%, Wolffi in 15.5% and Pomona in 6.7%. In the state of Amazonas, 880 bovine serum samples were analyzed, with Hardjo also occurring more frequently at 30.2%, followed by Wolffi at 22.4% and Bataviae at 6.0%.

Table 2 - Demonstration of *Leptospira spp.* serovars isolated in domestic animals in Brazil (Vasconcellos, personal communication, 2003).

Animal species	Sorovar	Author	Year	Source material
Canine	Icterohaemorrhagiae	Guida	1948	Kidney
Canine	Canicola	Guida	1948	Kidney
Swine	Guidae	Guida	1948	Kidney
Bovine	Pomona	Freitas *et al.*	1957	Fetus
Swine	Canicola	Guida *et al.*	1959	Fetus
Bovine	Icterohaemorrhagiae	Santa Rosa *et al.*	1961	Fetus
Swine	Guidae	Santa Rosa *et al.*	1962	Kidney
Swine	Icterohaemorrhagiae	Santa Rosa *et al.*	1962	Kidney
Swine	Pomona	Santa Rosa *et al.*	1962	Urine
Swine	Pomona	Santa Rosa *et al.*	1962	Kidney
Swine	Canicola	Castro *et al.*	1962	Kidney
Canine	Icterohaemorrhagiae	Castro *et al.*	1962	Kidney/Urine
Swine	Pomona	Santa Rosa *et al.*	1966	Fetus
Cattle	Guaicurus	Santa Rosa *et al.*	1967	Kidney

Swine	Icterohaemorrhagiae	Santa Rosa *et al.*	1970	Fetus
Swine	Pomona	Santa Rosa *et al.*	1970	Fetus
Bovine	Goiano	Santa Rosa *et al.*	1970	Kidney
Swine	Pomona	Cordeiro *et al.*	1973	Kidney
Canine	Canicola	Yasuda	1979	Kidney
Canine	Copenhageni	Yasuda	1979	Kidney
Canine	Pomona	Yasuda	1979	Kidney
Swine	Pomona	Oliveira *et al.*	1980	Fetus
Swine	Pomona	Oliveira *et al.*	1983	Kidney
Bovine	Hardjo	Moreira	1994	Urine
Bovine	Georgia	Moreira	1994	Urine
Bubalina	Guaricura	Vasconcellos *et al.*	2001	Urine

Homem (1999) analyzed properties with bovine herds in the municipality of Uruarà, in the state of Parà, and found 97% of properties with at least one animal positive for SAM, and in 61.2% of the herds the Hardjo serovar was indicated as the most likely, in 9% of them the Bratislava serovar and in 4.5% the Shermani serovar.

Negrao (1999) analyzed 417 samples from 23 cattle herds in Parà, 65.9% of which were positive, with Hardjo reacting in 20.1%, followed by Hebdomadis with 18.2%, Djasiman with 14.4%, Bratislava with 10.5%, Andamana with 7.1%, Patoc with 6.9% and Sejroe with 6.7%. The presence of leptospires was also demonstrated in kidney samples by silver impregnation, with a positivity rate of 34.7%. The demonstration of leptospires by Vàgó staining in urine and kidney samples showed 29.9% and 24.4% positivity, respectively.

Molnar *et al.* (2000) analyzed 131 cattle from seven herds in the state of Parà by SAM and ELISA and found a seropositivity rate of 74.7% in each test.

Negrao *et al.* (2001) analyzed 332 cattle and 345 buffalo and found 40.36% and 38.26% positivity, respectively. The serovar with the highest prevalence in both species was Hardjo with 29.85% and 31.81% of the positive samples from cattle and buffalo. The other serovars that reacted in cattle were: Patoc (17.16%), Hebdomadis (16.41%) and Wolffi (11.94%). The most reactive serovars in buffalo were Butembo (17.42%), Castellonis (12.87%), Autumnalis (10.60%) and Pomona (9.09%). Seropositive animals were found in all herds.

Negrao *et al.* (2002) analyzed 811 buffalo serum samples using two serological techniques, SAM and MAR, which showed 45.49% and 48.21% positivity, respectively. The percentage of positives in both tests was 26.75%. The serovars that reacted were Hardjo (52.84%), Autumnalis (15.71%), Wolffi (12.73%), Pomona (11.11%), Bratislava (7.85%), Butembo (7.58%), Castellonis (7.04%) and Patoc (5.14%).

Negrao *et al.* (2003) analyzed 811 serum samples from buffaloes from August 2000 to August 2002, and 377 samples from September 2002 to March 2003, and found 45.49% and 85.94% reagents, respectively. The most frequent serovars were Hardjo in the first period and Butembo in the second, and they concluded the high endemicity of Butembo and Hardjo with titers of up to 400 in the Pará herds surveyed.

1.5 Pathogenesis

Leptospira enters the body through abrasions of the skin and mucous membranes. After the incubation period of four to ten days, there is the bacteremia phase which can last seven days (Ellis, 1994), where there is intense multiplication in various organs, mainly the liver, spleen and kidneys, and by the fourth day there will be Ieptospira in the latter (Corrêa & Corrêa, 1992). This phase can be subclinical, but can also be characterized by pyrexia and anorexia, in which bacteria can be isolated from many organs (Ellis, 1994).

After this period, specific circulating antibodies appear, which are capable of opsonizing leptospires and are detectable from approximately the tenth day after infection begins (Ellis & McDowell, 1993). They persist for weeks or months, and in some cases for years. Unfortunately, antibody titres are often undetectable in chronically infected animals (OIE, 2001). Peak titres and the length of time they persist vary greatly depending on the animal species, the infecting serovar and the route of infection (Ellis & McDowell, 1993; Ellis, 1994).

Leptospires localize and persist especially in the proximal renal tubules. In infected cattle, they can remain in the female genital tract, mammary glands and male genital tract (Ellis *et al.,* 1985; Ellis & Thiermann, 1986; Ellis *et al.,* 1986; Bolin et *al.,* 1991). They are capable of multiplying in the pregnant uterus and in the lactating mammary gland and producing abortion and/or mastitis (Blood *et al.*, 1991).

Leptospiral infection persists for up to 142 days in the gravid uterus, 97 days in the non-gravid uterus and 83 days in the placenta and cotyledons (Thiermann, 1982). Ellis (1984) states that leptospires are excreted in uterine secretions for eight days and persist in the fallopian tubes for 22 days after birth. Ellis *et al.* (1986) isolated the Hardjo serovar from the testicle, epididymis and seminal vesicle of bulls, but with an unknown persistence period of infection.

1.6 Symptomatology

In animals, leptospirosis can present in various clinical forms and depends on the infecting serovar, the age of the animal and the physiological condition such as pregnancy and/or lactation (Ellis, 1994). In cattle, the vast majority of manifestations are subclinical and inapparent, and are capable of compromising the animal's reproductive efficiency, leading to infertility (Ellis & McDowell, 1993; Chaudhry *et al.,* 1996).

In beef herds, the primary economic loss due to leptospirosis is abortion (South & Stoenner, 1974). There is evidence that beef herds are more positive than dairy breeds (Miller *et al.,* 1991; Vasconcellos *et al.,* 1997). According to Vasconcellos *et al.* (1997), there is a greater association between heat repetitions and positivity than abortions and positivity.

In dairy herds, it is estimated that up to 30% of milk production is lost due to subclinical mastitis with a flaccid udder and yellowish milk with streaks of blood (Ellis & McDowell, 1993). Quinlan & McNicholl (1993) found a first calving conception rate of 49% in a herd with an agalactia epidemic.

In addition to reproductive disorders, cows that deliver their calves at term are born small and weak, and can die within the first few months of life, thus increasing the economic losses caused by leptospirosis in cattle herds (Ellis, 1994).

Miscarriage can occur at any stage of pregnancy, usually between one and twelve weeks after the acute phase. This depends not only on the serovar involved but also on the stage of pregnancy at the time of infection. Usually, 20 to 40% of cows abort when the infection occurs in the last trimester of pregnancy. After abortion, antibody titration is insignificant, often with a negative response to the microscopic serum agglutination test (Ellis & McDowell, 1993). Hardjo abortion occurs more frequently in the 3rd and 4th month of pregnancy, and the antibody titre decreases and can be below 100 (Genovez, 1999).

The most severe forms caused by accidental serovars are seen in calves with septicemia leading to pyrexia, anorexia, acute hemolytic anemia, hemoglobinuria and jaundice, which is often fatal. In adult animals there are abortions, stillbirths, lactation stops or the milk becomes pink and flakes of blood. Abortions occur one to six weeks after acute illness and high antibody titres are found (Ellis, 1994).

1.7 Diagnosis

The diagnosis of leptospirosis relies on the integration of clinical and epidemiological information with the results of laboratory tests. As the infection often has poor clinical symptoms or an inapparent form, clinical diagnosis becomes difficult and is therefore based solely on the results of laboratory procedures. These comprise two groups: the first consists of methods for demonstrating leptospires by direct research and the second are indirect methods for detecting leptospiral antibodies, serological tests (Ellis & McDowell, 1993), and definitive confirmation of infection is only possible through one of these parameters (Faine, 1982).

1.7.1. Direct methods for demonstrating leptospires

1.7.1.1. Isolation of leptospires in culture media

Leptospira isolation techniques are helpful in epidemiological studies, as the antibody titers investigated by serological tests are often undetectable in chronically infected animals (OIE, 2001). Isolating the bacteria from kidney carriers is very useful in epidemiological studies to determine which serovars are present in an animal species, a group of animals or a geographical location (Thiermann, 1984; Ellis & McDowell, 1993). Despite being a definitive diagnosis of leptospirosis, bacteriological cultures are often expensive, fresh samples are required and can take four to six months to complete, and are evaluated in specialized laboratories and reference centers, although isolation allows for certain identification of the infecting serovar (Bolin *et al.,* 1989).

Leptospires can be isolated by growth in culture media or inoculation in laboratory animals. Isolation depends on certain precautions in the bacteriological technique and some factors linked to it, such as the appropriate culture medium, alkaline pH (7.2 to 7.6), quality of the material collected and adequate cleaning of the glassware (Santa Rosa, 1970).

Two types of culture media are used for the growth of leptospires, depending on the purpose of the isolation: liquid and semi-solid media (University of Belgrade, 1997; OIE, 2001). The most widely used is the Ellinghausen & McCullough liquid medium, modified by Johnson & Harris (EMJH). It is essential for the growth of reference strains to be used as antigen for the serological test of microscopic serum agglutination, with weekly rechecks, and also for isolation from suspect material (Santa Rosa, 1970).

The semi-solid media are: EMJH medium plus 0.1 to 0.5% agar and Fletcher's medium. They are used for isolating strains from heavily contaminated material and take longer for the leptospires to grow. Fletcher's medium is also widely used to store strains for a longer period of time, requiring rechecks every six months. Despite being more expensive, this medium has an advantage over other semi-solid media because it is rich in proteins and is generally used when it is necessary to maintain the survival of leptospires for a longer period than EMJH (OIE, 2001).

Leptospires are unable to use amino acids or carbohydrates as important sources of energy, using long-chain fatty acids (Jawetz *et al.,* 1991) or enriching supplements purchased from appropriate laboratories. The media prepared in this way is incubated at 28° to 30°C for six weeks or more, and examined weekly under a darkfield microscope for up to two months, where it is considered negative if there is no morphology and movements characteristic of leptospires (Ministry of Health, 1995).

For the isolation of leptospires from suspected contaminated material, the medium used must be supplemented with antibiotics, as this eliminates contaminants that inhibit the proper growth of the leptospires. The most widely used antimicrobial is 5-fluorouracil, which, because it is a purimidic base, is not absorbed by leptospires, which only absorb bases that are pure to their nucleic acid (University of Belgrade, 1997). Other antimicrobials used are neomycin sulphate and nalidixic acid (Passos *et al.,* 1988).

Inoculation of laboratory animals is very useful for isolating leptospires. They can also serve as a means of maintaining strains that do not adapt well to culture media. The laboratory species used in the routine diagnosis of leptospirosis are hamsters and guinea pigs. Young animals, preferably weaned, should be used for isolation (Santa Rosa, 1970).

1.7.1.2. Molecular Methods

The presence of leptospires in organic material can be confirmed by identifying the bacterium's nucleic acid. Various molecular methodology techniques are being used to demonstrate the causative agent of leptospirosis (Deacon & Lah, 1999).

At the end of the 1980s, the technique that would revolutionize the study of DNA, the Polymerase Chain Reaction (PCR), was described. Unlike the techniques previously used, the new technique was very fast and simple to carry out (Pires, 2002). These methods require equipped laboratories and personnel trained in the methodology of molecular genetics (Woodward *et al.,* 1997), but can provide rapid and sensitive diagnosis (Smith *et al.,* 1994). The specificity of the test can be related to the knowledge of a part of the leptospira genome (conserved sequence) or its related group, however, when it is restricted to the serovar level, its specificity is greater (Prado, 1999).

To start sequencing, the polymerase enzyme adds nucleotides to the sequence of a matrix molecule. This enzyme needs a support point (sequence of nucleotides already bound to this molecule). The sequence of 20 to 30 nucleotides that will bind to each of the helices, delimiting the fragment to be copied, is called a *primer. The* DNA molecule with its separate helices and each specific *primer* will be copied and duplicated (Van Eys *et al.,* 1991, Smith *et al.,* 1994; Pires, 2002).

The *primers* are the initiators for duplicating the sequence to form the 3' and 5' portions, producing an exponential copy of the selected sequence. The products are detected either by hybridization or by direct observation after a run of gel electrophoresis stained with ethidium bromide. A minimum of two pairs of *primers* are required, which are contained in the 3' and 5' base pair (bp) portions of a specific leptospira nucleic acid sequence. These *primers* are differentiated by the direction in which the nucleotide sequence will bind to the nucleic acid (Prado, 1999).

Mérien *et al.* (1992) developed a PCR technique that is capable of demonstrating *Leptospira sp.* A 331 bp sequence of the rrs (16S) gene of *Leptospira interrogans* serovar Canicola was amplified, and the PCR analyzed by DNA-DNA hybridization using the internal fragment of 289 bp. Specific products were also obtained with *L. biflexa* DNA, but not with the DNA of other spirochetes or other organisms such as *Escherichia coli, Staphylococcus aureus, Mycobacterium tuberculosis and Proteus mirabilis.* The lowest detection limit was less than 10 bacteria.

Romero *et al.* (1998) tested PCR, ELISA-IgM and SAM on 103 cerebrospinal fluid samples from human patients with meningitis of unknown origin. This study showed that 39.80% were positive by PCR, while 3.88% and 8.74% were positive by ELISA-IgM and SAM, respectively.

Heinemann *et al.* (2000) detected by PCR the serovars Andamana, Brasiliensis, Buenos Aires, Butembo, Garcia, Rufino and Whitcombi from experimentally infected bovine semen samples in Brazil, and showed that PCR has great potential for detecting leptospires in semen samples from bulls kept in artificial insemination centers.

1.7.2. Indirect methods of demonstrating leptospires

1.7.2.1. Microscopic Serum Agglutination Test (SAM)

SAM is the basis for the diagnosis and classification of leptospires and is therefore the most widely used serological test for the diagnosis of leptospirosis, being the standard serological test, or reference test, against all other diagnostic tests used (OIE, 2001) and being serogroup-specific (Ellis & McDowell, 1993). It is also the most widely used test to confirm the clinical diagnosis of the disease, to determine the prevalence of herds and to conduct epidemiological studies (Ellis & McDowell, 1993).

It has optimum sensitivity because it involves live antigens and reference strains of serovars that represent all the known serogroups in the region or animal species being tested. The presence of the serogroup is usually indicated by frequent reactions in the sera tested or by isolating the serovar from infected animals. The sensitivity of the test can be increased by including locally isolated strains in the battery of serovars evaluated (OIE, 2001).

The specificity of SAM is high, as antibodies against other bacteria usually do not cross-react with *Leptospira.* However, there are significant cross-reactions between *Leptospira* serovars, and an animal infected with one serovar probably has antibodies against it, but may cross-react with other serovars, and usually has low levels of antibodies detectable in the SAM (Ellis & McDowell, 1993; OIE, 2001).

This method has been standardized over the last century by various researchers, who have taken into account factors such as: ideal incubation time and temperature, reading, cut-off point, titration, density and age of the cultures. These studies resulted in the definition of the SAM with different purposes used today, which are defined as a serial dilution of the serum to be tested, in contact with an equal volume of leptospira growth suspension, at a certain temperature, for a certain period of time and read, under microscopy, considering the final titre, the dilution that agglutinates 50% or more of the leptospires (Korver, 2000).

The use of SAM is primarily as a herd test. As an individual animal test, SAM is very useful for diagnosing acute infection when there are paired serum samples from the acute and convalescent phases (Ellis & McDowell, 1993). Its methodology uses live antigens, with strains representing all the serogroups that occur in the region or country. It is based on the phenomenon of agglutination of surface antigen components present in living organisms or lysis of the bacteria (OIE, 2001).

It often shows reactions to more than one serovar (in a single serological sample analyzed), because the antigens used are live leptospira strains representing various serovars. It is known that the outer membrane of the leptospira has a great diversity of antigenic components and that these elements combine with the antibodies present in the sera tested, causing an antigen-antibody agglutination reaction. This can lead to cross-reactions between different serovars belonging to the same serogroup (homologous) and even between serovars belonging to different serogroups (heterologous). These reactions are most commonly found in the first few weeks of the disease, causing a phenomenon called the "paradoxical reaction" (Korver, 2000). It is therefore necessary to evaluate the serological results at serovar level and the final titres found in the entire herd, in order to characterize the infecting serogroup and the most likely serovar to cause the disease (Vasconcellos *et al.,* 1997).

Accepted worldwide, the antibody levels considered positive in the SAM test, in infections by any serovar, are titers of 100 or higher. The disadvantage of considering a higher titer as a cut-off point for positivity, for example 200, is that it is possible to underestimate the positivity of animals with a lower level of antibodies, or to increase the percentage of susceptible animals in the herd. Similarly, if the cut-off point were a 1:50 dilution (titer 50), we would have exaggerated numbers of false positives and consequently underestimate the percentage of susceptible animals in the herd (Korver, 2000; OIE, 2001).

In vaccinated animals, vaccine titers are only differentiated by SAM when there is paired serology, where the initial antibodies are short-lived and the antibodies formed later (from 15 days apart) are longer-lived and have higher values (Dhaliwal *et al.,* 1996).

SAM has limitations in the diagnosis of chronic infections in individual animals, both in the diagnosis of abortion and in the identification of renal and genital carriers. Infected animals often have low or no detectable titer by SAM when infected with Bratislava in pigs and Hardjo in cattle and sheep (Thiermann & Garrett, 1983).

1.7.2.2. Rapid macroagglutination plate test (MAR)

This test uses concentrated and standardized suspensions of inactivated leptospires that are stable for one year. It is indicated for screening, as it provides quick results and is easy to perform, being widely used in the screening of human sera (Ministry of Health, 1995).

It has the advantage of showing antibodies earlier than SAM. For the examination of past infections and the search for residual antibodies, it is less sensitive than SAM. Another disadvantage is that it does not show the infecting serogroup (Santa Rosa, 1970).

Caldas *et al.* (1997) obtained excellent results comparing the LEPTOTEST (macroagglutination, developed by the Osvaldo Cruz Foundation - RJ) with the SAM, citing high sensitivity and precocity, with the aim of being adopted by professionals at field level and by small laboratories.

1.8 Control and Treatment

Controlling leptospirosis depends mainly on knowing which serovars are reactive in the region. This makes it necessary to vaccinate and even treat the animals. These disease control measures are of the utmost importance, since leptospirosis is an endemic disease that is difficult to eradicate, as many animal species (including wild ones) act as hosts, spreading the leptospira in the environment (Vasconcellos, 1987).

Vaccination with leptospiral bacterins is the most effective method for controlling leptospirosis (Ellis & McDowell, 1993). Most vaccines are formalin-inactivated bacterins and are specific to the serovars prevalent in a region, with specific immunity for each serovar (Vasconcellos *et al.,* 1997).

Vaccination does not stop infection in an Ieptospira animal, and does not always prevent abortion if the animal has been infected before, leading to localization of the leptospira in the placenta. It also does not necessarily prevent leptospirosis, despite the good immune response, and is not completely efficient in preventing new cases of infection when there is a high level of natural challenge, however, this decreases as the animals are vaccinated, increasing the level of control in the herd (Genovez *et al.,* 2003).

Treatment consists of administering a single dose of 25mg/kg of dihydrostreptomycin (Ellis & McDowell, 1993) and Gallego & Gallego (1994) recommend two doses of 25 mg/kg, administered at 7-day intervals. Faine (1982) recommends a dose of 11mg/kg, every 12 hours for 3 days, or 5g twice for 3 consecutive days, which can be effective in curing the acute phase and eliminating the carrier state. Gallego & Gallego (1994) admit that a dose of 25mg/kg for 3 days is 90% effective in chronically infected cows.

Vaccination together with treatment with dihydrostreptomycin (25mg/kg, once) effectively combats the infection, along with other management measures (Ellis & McDowell, 1993).

Other management practices can be taken to reduce the risk factors for a herd: separating acquired animals from the rest of the herd (quarantine), controlling the access of infected animals to rivers or lakes (separation of sick and suspect animals) and not allowing breeding with pigs and sheep (Bennett, 1991 and 1993).

Acquired animals that are isolated should be treated with streptomycin and vaccinated before joining the controlled herd (Ellis & McDowell, 1993). Another advisable practice would be the regular serology (every 6 months) of 10% of the herd, thus allowing the health situation of the disease to be mapped (Faine, 1982).

1.9 Public Health

In addition to its economic importance, animal leptospirosis is even more important from a public health point of view, as human infections can be acquired from sick animals and/or carriers (FUNASA, 2003).

Man acquires the infection through contact with animals or through the urine of contaminated animals. It is considered to be an accidental zoonosis, with an occupational risk for farmers, veterinarians, ranchers, animal handlers and garbage collectors (Ellis & McDowell, 1993). Contact can be direct or more often indirect, through contamination of infected urine and also through uterine contents (Ellis & McDowell, 1993). However, the disease can be acquired in other situations, such as through recreation. Almeida *et al.* (1994) state that leptospirosis is associated more with recreational activities than with occupational diseases. Garcia & Navarro (2001) found a significant difference in relation to patients who reported having helped deliver animals. They found no statistical difference between individuals who consumed raw or undercooked meat, raw milk or simple contact with animals.

In Brazil, there are many epidemiological inquiries into human leptospirosis, the vast majority of which correspond to transmission from rodents and dogs, involving the serovars Icterohaemorrhagiae, Australis, Copenhageni, Pomona, Tarassovi, Canicola and others, depending on the region (Corrêa & Corrêa, 1992).

Mackintosh *et al.* (1982) reported that the risk of animal handlers contracting Hardjo's infection is directly proportional to the endemicity of the herd, while the risk of Pomona is related to the introduction of new animals and the breeding of pigs close to the herd.

2. Objectives

2.1. General

To demonstrate *Leptospira spp,* through direct and indirect diagnostic methods, in buffaloes destined for slaughter and coming from the micro-region of Arari, Marajó Archipelago, State of Parà.

2.2. Specifics

1. To demonstrate the seroprevalence of leptospirosis, using SAM, in buffaloes from the Arari micro-region, Marajó Archipelago.

2. To demonstrate the prevalence of serological variants of *Leptospira spp* in buffalo herds, using SAM.

3. Discriminate the seroprevalence of leptospirosis in the municipalities of the Arari micro-region, Marajó Archipelago, using SAM.

4. Discriminate the seroprevalence of leptospirosis according to the sex of the animals, using the SAM.

5. Research into the presence of *Leptospira spp* strains, using the technique of isolating the agent in culture media, in kidney and urine samples from buffaloes in the Arari micro-region.

6. To correlate the serological variant found, using SAM, in animals that tested positive by isolating the agent in culture medium, in kidney and/or urine samples from buffaloes in the Arari micro-region.

7. To examine the possibility of MAR as a serological screening test for leptospirosis in buffaloes, by correlating it with SAM positivity.

8. To use the PCR technique as a serovar-specific test for *Leptospira interrogans* serovar Hardjo in kidney and urine samples from Marajoa buffaloes.

3. Materials and methods

3.1. MATERIALS

3.1.1. Herds and animals

We evaluated 10 buffalo herds from 10 rural properties located in the municipalities of the Arari micro-region, belonging to the Marajó meso-region, in the state of Parà (Figure 2).

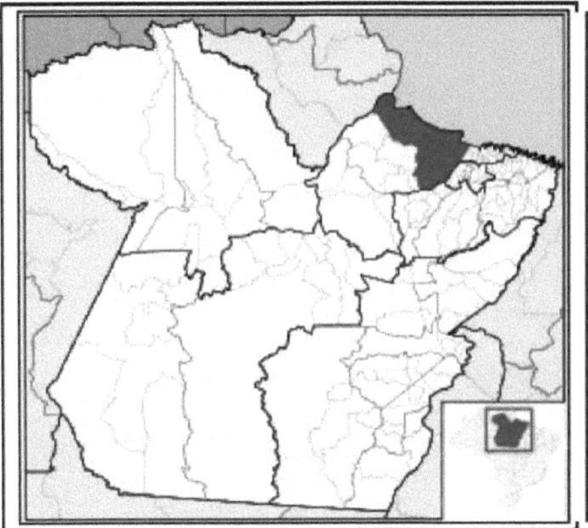

Figure 2 - Illustrative map of the mesoregions of the state of Parà, highlighting the Arari microregion belonging to the Marajó mesoregion (Wikipedia, 2006).

The herds included were chosen on the basis of prior knowledge of the municipality of origin, zootechnical and sanitary conditions, age and sex of the animals (information provided by those responsible for the farms via telephone call). All the herds belonged to rural properties with a similar zootechnical and health profile, representative of the reality of most Marajoaras herds.

The type of livestock farming was extensive, with a herd of over 200 head. The only immunization practice adopted was vaccination against foot-and-mouth disease twice a year. The animals sent for slaughter were over 36 months old. The properties of origin were home to free-living wild animals such as: neo-tropical primates (*Cebus apella, Leontopithecus sp., Saguinus sp., Saimiri sp.*), paca (*Agouti paca),* armadillo (*Dasypus novemcintus*), sloth (*Bradypus infuscatus*), caimans (*Caiman sp),* caititu (*Tayassu tajacu*), tortoises (*Geochelone carbonaria)* and birds in general. The most common reproductive disorders described by those responsible were increased calving intervals and infertility, cited by the breeders as the delay in females becoming pregnant or never becoming pregnant. Abortion was seen occasionally on the farms.

The number of herds sampled per municipality was directly related to the number of buffalo herds in the region, according to data from the 2005 Municipal Livestock Survey (IBGE, 2005). As the

Arari micro-region has seven municipalities, three herds were sampled from Chaves and two from Cachoeira do Arari. The other five herds belonged to one municipality each.

Figure 3 illustrates the municipalities sampled and discriminates the number of herds studied by the color of the symbol in the figure, with red representing three herds; blue, two herds and green, one herd in each municipality.

Each herd studied was catalogued according to its municipality of origin. From each municipality, 20 animals were sampled, totaling 10 herds, resulting in 200 animals. Of these herds, five were males and five were females.

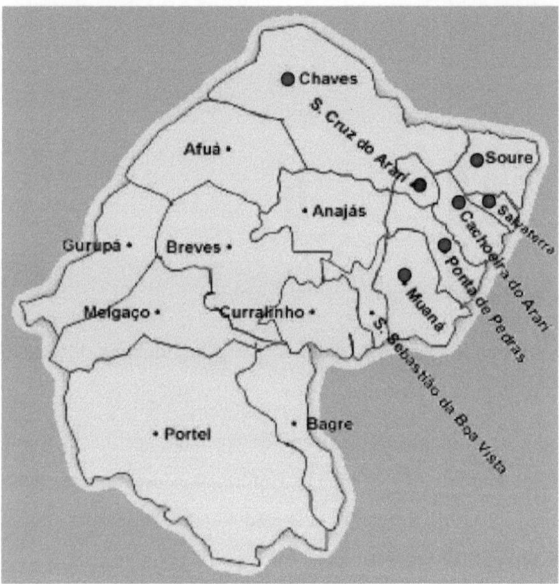

Figure 3 - Illustrative map of the Marajó mesoregion, highlighting the municipalities of the Arari microregion (Wikipedia, 2006).

Biological material was collected between August 2003 and May 2005. Data such as sex, municipality of origin and month/year of collection for each herd are shown in Table 3.

3.1.2. Sample collection site

The biological samples were collected at the SOCIPE (Sociedade Cooperativa da Indùstria Pecuària do Parà) slaughterhouse, which is registered with the State Inspection Service (SIE) and is located in the district of Icoaracy, in the municipality of Belém.

Table 3. Data on buffalo herds from the municipalities from which the biological samples were taken.

Flock	Sex	City of origin	Harvest month and year
1	Female	Keys	August/2003
2	Female	Keys	October/2003
3	Male	Arari Waterfall	December/2003
4	Male	Soure	March/2004
5	Male	Santa Cruz do Arari	May/2004
6	Male	Ponta de Pedras	August/2004
7	Female	Salvaterra	October/2004
8	Female	Muanà	December/2004
9	Male	Keys	March 2005
10	Female	Arari Waterfall	May/2005

3.1.3. Samples

Blood, urine and kidney samples were collected from the same animal. Blood samples were taken from all 200 animals, but urine and kidney samples were taken from five animals in each herd. At the slaughterhouse, the order of animals sampled from each herd was determined by the first 20 animals lined up in the corridor of the stunning box. The five animals chosen for kidney and urine collection from each herd were determined randomly, with an interval of every five animals for collection.

All the samples were sent to the Laboratory for the Investigation and Diagnosis of Animal Diseases (LIDEA) at the Agricultural Center of the Federal University of Pará. An aliquot of the urine and kidney samples, intended for PCR processing, were stored and kept at minus 20° C until they were transported in an isothermal box with ice to the Biological Institute Laboratory in Sao Paulo - SP, where they were processed.

3.1.3.1. Blood serum

Blood samples were collected in sterile 20 mL test tubes when the animal was bled at the slaughterhouse. In the laboratory, the blood was dried and the serum stored in *eppendorf* microtubes at minus 20° C until the serological tests were carried out. The blood serum samples were used for the SAM and MAR serological tests.

3.1.3.2. Urine

A Bunsen burner was used at all stages of urine collection and seeding in the slaughterhouse to reduce the possibility of contamination. Urine samples were collected directly from the bladder, previously aseptically with iodized alcohol, by puncture with a sterile, disposable needle and syringe, in an approximate quantity of 5 mL, according to the protocol described by Ellis *et al.* (1986). These samples were used for leptospira isolation and PCR.

1. Samples for Isolation

0.5 mL of urine was sown in 5 mL of selective EMJH medium, to a final dilution of 10^{-1} (1:10 or the ratio of one part urine to nine parts culture medium) and transported to the laboratory at room temperature, according to the protocol of Heinemann *et al.* (2000).

2. Samples for PCR

2 mL were placed in sterile, capped test tubes and transported to the laboratory in an isothermal box with ice. In the laboratory, the samples were stored in *epipeiidorf-type* microtubes and stored at minus 20° C for PCR processing.

3.1.3.3. Kidney

Two kidney lobules were collected from each animal, packed in a plastic bag and transported to the laboratory in an isothermal box with ice, according to the protocol described by Ellis *et al.* (1986). Of this material, one kidney lobe was used to isolate the agent and the other was kept at minus 20° C for PCR processing.

3.2. . METHODS

3.2.1. Microscopic Serum Agglutination Test (SAM)

This test was carried out as recommended by Santa Rosa (1970).

a) Antigen

Live antigens were used from cultures of laboratory strains of *Leptospira,* maintained in EMJH medium plus 10% enrichment (*Leptospira enrichment* EMJH - DIFCO) from cultures repeated weekly, and kept in a bacteriological incubator at 28°C. All antigens were used on the sixth day of incubation. A collection of 25 strains representing the most epidemiologically important serovars in cattle in Brazil was used (23 pathogenic strains and two saprophytes) (Table 4).

Table 4 - List of *Leptospira* serovars used as antigens in the microscopic serum agglutination test, according to species, serogroup and serovar (Ellis, 1995).

Species	Serogroup	Sorovar
	Australis	Australis

		Bratislava
	Autumnalis	Autumnalis
		Butembo
	Bataviae	Bataviae
	Canicola	Canicola
	Celedoni	Whitcombi
L. interrogans	Djasiman	Sensot
	Hebdomadis	Hebdomadis
	Pomona	Pomona
	Icterohaemorrhagi ae	Icterohaemorrhagiae
		Copenhageni
	Pyrogenes	Pyrogenes
	Cynopteri	Cynopteri
	Sejroe	Hardj o
		Wolffi
	Ballum	Castellonis
	Javanica	Javanica
L. borgpetersenii	Mini	Mini
	Tarassovi	Tarassovi
L. noguchii	Panama	Panama
L. santarosai	Shermani	Shermani
L. kirsheneri	Grippotyphosa	Grippotyphosa
	Andamana	Andamana
L. biflexa	Semaranga	Patoc

The antigens were checked both macroscopically and microscopically in order to determine density, purity and possible self-agglutination that could lead to errors in the reading. The macroscopic control was carried out by observing with the naked eye the slight opalescence in the culture medium, in which the movement resembling "cigarette smoke" was observed when the tube was shaken slightly.

For microscopic examination, a drop of the culture was placed on a slide covered with laminate, and the characteristic movement of the leptospires and the presence or absence of other bacteria were observed under a microscope using a darkfield condenser with a 10x objective and eyepiece.

b) Soros controls

The respective bovine blood sera known to be positive and negative for each serovar were used as positive and negative controls. The control for each strain was also used.

c) Test procedure

Initially, each serum was screened at a dilution of 1:50 in TSS. To do this, 50 μL of the diluted serum was added and 50 μL of antigen was added, leaving a titration of 100. The plate was then placed in an oven at 37 C for two hours.

d) Reading

It was carried out under a microscope using a dark field condenser with a 10x objective and eyepiece, by observing a drop of each serum tested on a glass microscope slide, covered with a coverslip. The degree of agglutination observed could be 1+ (25% of leptospires agglutinated), 2+ (50% agglutinated), 3+ (75% agglutinated) or 4+ (100% agglutinated or lysed), with only those above 2+ being considered positive. The serum tested that showed a reduction in the number of free leptospires in the order of 50 to 100% compared to the control was submitted to the titration test.

e) Titration

It was diluted 1:200 in SST with consecutive titrations and doubled up to 6,400. Then 50μL of the corresponding antigen was added to each serum tested. Positive, negative and antigen controls were also added. The highest dilution of serum capable of agglutinating 50% or more of the leptospires compared to the control was considered the final titre (Leptospirosis Manual, 1995).

f) Analysis of results

The serovar with the highest titer and the highest number of positive animals in the herd was considered the most likely (Vasconcellos *et al.,* 1997).

3.2.2. Rapid Macroagglutination Test (MAR)

This test was standardized by the Oswaldo Cruz Foundation - Bio-Manguinhos for the diagnosis of human leptospirosis called LEPTOTEST.

a) Antigen

An antigenic suspension produced from a *pool* of inactivated and standardized Ieptospira was used.

b) Test procedure

Ten μL of each serum tested was added to 55 μL of the antigen and homogenized with a rod. Oscillatory movements were then made on the plate for 10 seconds before it was vortexed for 4 minutes at 125 revolutions per minute. Positive and negative controls were also added.

c) Reading

An indirect light source was used against a dark background. The test samples were compared with the controls. The presence of lumps in unclear medium was considered a positive reaction and the absence of lumps in opalescent medium a negative reaction.

3.2.3. Isolation of Leptospires

This technique was carried out according to the protocols of Faine (1982) and Santa Rosa (1970).

a) Culture media

The culture media used for the isolation of leptospires were EMJH and modified EMJH liquid media and Fletcher's semi-solid medium. EMJH liquid medium and Fletcher's semi-solid medium were prepared according to the manufacturer (BECTON DICKINSON). The modified EMJH medium is the selective medium for growing leptospires (EMJH with antibiotics) according to the protocol of Heinemann *et al.* (2000) and Miraglia *et al.* (2003), and includes the addition of the antimicrobials 5-fluorouracil 300mg/L of EMJH medium and nalidixic acid 20mg/L of EMJH medium.

b) Cultivation procedures

1. Urine

Using the initial dilution of 1:10 ($10^{\wedge 1}$) made when the sample was taken, serial dilutions of 1:100 and 1:1,000 were made, corresponding respectively to the dilutions 10^{-2} and 10^{-3} . Of these dilutions, 0.5 mL were sown in 5 mL of the selective medium plus antibiotics, which remained for 24 hours at a temperature of 28° to 30° C. After this period, the cultures were replanted in EMJH medium without antibiotics, at a temperature of 28° to 30^0 C. These cultures were observed weekly for eight weeks. An attempt was made to visualize the subsurface growth ring and, if positive, confirmation was made by microscopic examination to verify the presence of leptospires. After this period, the negative cultures were discarded. Those cultures that showed positive growth for leptospires were repeated in Fletcher's medium.

2. Kidney

A fragment of the inside of the organ (approximately one gram) was collected and ground with a sterile grater and pistil (one gram of tissue for 9 mL of TSS). Serial dilutions of 1:10, 1:100 and

1:1,000 (10^{-1}, 10^{-2} and 10^{-3}) were then prepared, as with the urine samples. 0.5 mL of these dilutions were also sown in 5 mL of the selective medium plus antibiotics, and left for 24 hours at a temperature of 28° to 30° C. After this period, the cultures were repeated in EMJH medium without antibiotics, at a temperature of 28° to 30° C.

These cultures were observed weekly for eight weeks. An attempt was made to visualize the subsurface growth ring and, if positive, confirmation was made by microscopic examination to verify the presence of leptospira. After this period, the negative cultures were discarded. Those cultures that showed positive growth for leptospires were repeated in Fletcher's medium.

3.2.4. Polymerase Chain Reaction (PCR)

It was carried out according to the protocols described by Mérien *et al.* (1992) and Scarcelli *et al.* (2000).

a) Sample preparation

The DNA was extracted in 1.5 mL tubes. The samples were centrifuged at 13,000 x g for 10 minutes. To the sediments, 400 µL of TE (TRIS-HCL 10 Mm, EDTA 1 Mm, pH 8.0) were added, vortexed for 10 seconds and centrifuged at 13,000 x g for 10 minutes. An aliquot of the sediment (100 µL) from each sample was processed according to the standard protocol of the DNA extraction kit "DNAzol reagent" (GIBCO-BRL). The DNA obtained was stored at -20° C. DNA extracted from a culture of *Leptospira interrogans* serovar Hardjo, strain Hardjoprajitno, was used as a positive control, and ultrapure water was used as a negative control.

b) DNA amplification

Gene-specific primer oligonucleotides (Lep 1 and lep 2) were used from the 16S rRNA gene sequence of *Leptospira interrogans* serovar Canicola, which amplify a 330 bp fragment: Lep 1: 5' GGC GGC GCG TCT TAA ACA TG 3' and Lep 2: 3' TTC CCC CCA TTG AGC AAG ATT 5'. Ten µL of extracted DNA was added to 21.2 µL of water, 5 µL of 10 X buffer (500 mM KCl, 15 mM $MgCl_2$, 100mM TRIS-HCl, pH 9.0), 1.5 µL of 50mM $MgCl_2$, 8 µL of dNTP mixture (200 mM of each nucleotide [dCTP, dATP, dGT, dTTP]), 4 µL of *primers* (Lep1 and lep 2 - pmol/mL of each), 0.5 µL of *Taq* DNA polymerase (5 units per µL).

The samples were first denatured at 95° C for five minutes, followed by 29 amplification cycles divided into four phases: 1 - Denaturation - 94° C/60 seconds; 2 - Ringing - 63° C/90 seconds; 3 - Extension - 72° C/120 seconds and 4 - Final extension - 72° C/10 minutes.

c) Analysis of the amplified product

It was carried out by electrophoresis on a 2.0% agarose gel with a 0.5 X TBE running buffer

(0.04M TRIS - borate and 1 mM EDTA, pH 8.0) and the gel subjected to a constant voltage of 6 - 7V/cm. The molecular weight standard used was 100 bp. The gel was stained with 0.5μg/mL ethidium bromide and then photographed under ultraviolet light (300-320 nm) using a photo-documentation system (Kodak Digital DC/120 Zoom camera) and analyzed using 1D Image Analysis software (Kodak Digital Science).

3.2.5. Statistical Method

The results of the two serological techniques used were statistically compared and determined using the Chi-Square test, using the Epi-Info 6.04 program, with a significance level of 0.05, considering SAM as the reference serological test recommended by the World Health Organization. The MAR parameters were those adopted by Caldas *et al.* (1997) and Medronho *et al.* (2002), using the following analysis:

S Determination of Sensitivity: number of animals positive for MAR that were also positive for SAM divided by the number of animals positive for SAM.

S Determination of Specificity: number of animals negative to both serological tests divided by the number of animals negative to SAM.

s Determination of false positives: number of MAR-negative animals divided by the number of SAM-negative animals.

s Determination of false-negatives: number of animals negative by MAR of those positive by SAM divided by the number of animals positive by SAM.

s Determination of MAR/SAM concordance: number of animals positive to both serological tests added to the number of animals negative to both tests and divided by the number of animals tested.

4. Results

The individual results of the diagnosis of Ieptospirosis in the Marajoara bubalinos analyzed are broken down by herd in Tables 1 to 10. All the herds tested positive for the two serological tests used (SAM and MAR). However, in the direct demonstration methods, not all the herds analyzed detected the etiological agent, since the isolation of leptospires was only demonstrated in six herds surveyed, while PCR was not possible in any of them.

Herd 1 was positive for SAM in 11 samples (Butembo and Hardjo); for MAR in 5 samples and 1 for renal isolation (Table 1). In herd 2, 10 samples reacted by SAM (Butembo, Hardjo, Pyrogenes and Shermani); 3 by MAR and 5 kidney and 3 urine samples (Table 2). Herd 3 reacted to 9 samples by SAM (Butembo and Autumnalis); 5 by MAR and 3 by renal isolation (Table 3). In herd 4, 15 samples reacted by SAM (Butembo and Hardjo); 4 by MAR and 1 by renal isolation (Tables 4). In herd 5, 9 samples reacted by SAM (Butembo only); 3 by MAR and none by isolation (Table 5). In herd 6, 11 samples reacted by SAM (Butembo and Autumnalis); 9 by MAR and 2 by renal isolation (Table 6). In herd 7, 15 samples reacted by SAM (Butembo, Hardjo and Pomona); 10 by MAR and 2 by renal isolation and 1 by urinary isolation (Table 7). In herd 8, 12 samples reacted by SAM (Hardjo, Pomona, Castellonis and Bratislava); 3 by MAR and none by isolation (Table 8). In herd 9, 8 samples reacted to SAM (Hardjo and Autumnalis); 6 to MAR and none to isolation (Table 9). In herd 10, 6 samples reacted by SAM (Butembo and Hardjo); 7 by MAR and none by isolation (Table 10).

Table 01. Demonstration of the diagnosis of leptospirosis in the biological samples analyzed, belonging to herd 1 and coming from the municipality of Chaves, according to the technique used, Belém, 2007.

Sample	SAM			MAR	Isolation	
	Results	Reactive serovar	Final title		Kidney	Urine
01	Positive	Butembo	100	Negative	Negative	Negative
02	Positive	Butembo	400	Positive	Negative	Negative
03	Negative	-	-	Negative	Negative	Negative
04	Positive	Hardj o	100	Negative	Negative	Negative
05	Negative	-	-	Negative	Negative	Negative
06	Positive	Butembo	100	Negative	Negative	Negative
07	Negative	-	-	Negative	Negative	Negative
08	Negative	-	-	Negative	Negative	Negative

09	Positive	Butembo	100	Negative	Negative	Negative
10	Positive	Butembo	100	Negative	Negative	Negative
11	Negative	-	-	Negative	Negative	Negative
12	Negative	-	-	Negative	Negative	Negative
13	Positive	Butembo	100	Positive	Negative	Negative
14	Negative	-	-	Positive	Negative	Negative
15	Positive	Butembo	100	Negative	Negative	Negative
16	Negative	-	-	Negative	Negative	Negative
17	Positive	Butembo	100	Positive	Negative	Negative
18	Negative	-	-	Negative	Negative	Negative
19	Positive	Butembo	100	Positive	Negative	Negative
20	Positive	Hardj o	100	Negative	Positive	Negative
Total	11	Butembo Hardj o	100, 400	5	1	0

Table 02. Demonstration of the diagnosis of Ieptospirosis in the biological samples analyzed, belonging to herd 2 and coming from the municipality of Chaves, according to the technique used, Belém, 2007.

Sample	SAM			MAR	Isolation	
	Results	Reactive serovar	Final title		Kidney	Urine
01	Positive	Hardj o	100	Negative	Positive	Negative
02	Negative	-	-	Negative	Negative	Negative
03	Negative	-	-	Negative	Negative	Negative
04	Negative	-	-	Negative	Negative	Negative
05	Positive	Hardj o	100	Negative	Negative	Positive
06	Negative	-	-	Negative	Negative	Negative
07	Positive	Pyrogenes	100	Negative	Negative	Negative
08	Positive	Butembo	200	Positive	Negative	Negative
09	Positive	Butembo	100	Negative	Negative	Negative
10	Positive	Butembo	100	Negative	Positive	Negative
11	Negative	-	-	Positive	Negative	Negative
12	Negative	-	-	Negative	Negative	Negative
13	Negative	-	-	Negative	Negative	Negative
14	Negative	-	-	Negative	Negative	Negative

15	Positive	Hardj o	100	Negative	Positive	Positive
16	Negative	-	-	Negative	Negative	Negative
17	Positive	Shermani	100	Positive	Negative	Negative
18	Positive	Butembo	200	Negative	Negative	Negative
19	Negative	-	-	Negative	Negative	Negative
20	Positive	Hardj o	100	Negative	Negative	Negative
Total	10	Butembo Hardjo Pyrogenes Shermani	100, 200	3	3	2

Table 03. Demonstration of the diagnosis of leptospirosis in the biological samples analyzed, belonging to herd 3 and coming from Cachoeira do Arari, according to the technique used, Belém, 2007.

Sample	SAM			MAR	Isolation	
	Results	Reactive serovar	Final title		Kidney	Urine
01	Positive	Autumnalis	100	Positive	Positive	Negative
02	Negative	-	-	Positive	Negative	Negative
03	Negative	-	-	Negative	Negative	Negative
04	Negative	-	-	Negative	Negative	Negative
05	Positive	Butembo	100	Positive	Positive	Negative
06	Negative	-	-	Negative	Negative	Negative
07	Negative	-	-	Negative	Negative	Negative
08	Positive	Butembo	100	Negative	Negative	Negative
09	Positive	Butembo	100	Positive	Negative	Negative
10	Negative	-	-	Positive	Negative	Negative
11	Positive	Butembo	100	Negative	Negative	Negative
12	Negative	-	-	Negative	Negative	Negative
13	Negative	-	-	Negative	Negative	Negative
14	Positive	Butembo	200	Negative	Negative	Negative
15	Negative	-	-	Negative	Negative	Negative
16	Positive	Butembo	100	Negative	Negative	Negative
17	Positive	Butembo	200	Negative	Negative	Negative
18	Negative	-	-	Negative	Negative	Negative

19	Negative	-	-	Negative	Negative	Negative
20	Positive	Butembo	100	Negative	Positive	Negative
Total	9	Autumnalis Butembo	100, 200	5	3	0

Table 4. Demonstration of the diagnosis of leptospirosis in the biological samples analyzed, belonging to herd 4 and coming from the municipality of Soure, according to the technique used, Belém, 2007.

Sample	SAM			- SEA	Isolation	
	Results	Reactive serovar	Final title		Kidney	Urine
01	Negative	-	-	Negative	Negative	Negative
02	Positive	Butembo	100	Negative	Negative	Negative
03	Positive	Butembo	100	Negative	Negative	Negative
04	Positive	Butembo	100	Negative	Negative	Negative
05	Positive	Hardj o	100	Negative	Positive	Negative
06	Negative	-	-	Negative	Negative	Negative
07	Positive	Hardjo	100	Negative	Negative	Negative
08	Positive	Butembo	100	Negative	Negative	Negative
09	Positive	Hardj o	100	Negative	Negative	Negative
10	Positive	Hardj o	100	Positive	Negative	Negative
11	Positive	Hardj o	100	Negative	Negative	Negative
12	Positive	Hardj o	100	Positive	Negative	Negative
13	Positive	Hardj o	100	Positive	Negative	Negative
14	Negative	-	-	Negative	Negative	Negative
15	Positive	Hardj o	100	Negative	Negative	Negative
16	Positive	Hardj o	100	Negative	Negative	Negative
17	Negative	-	-	Negative	Negative	Negative
18	Negative	-	-	Negative	Negative	Negative
19	Positive	Hardj o	100	Negative	Negative	Negative
20	Positive	Hardj o	100	Positive	Negative	Negative
Total	15	Butembo Hardj o	100	4	1	0

Table 5. Demonstration of the diagnosis of Ieptospirosis in the biological samples analyzed, belonging to herd 5 and coming from the municipality of Santa Cruz do Arari, according to the technique used, Belém, 2007.

Sample	SAM			MAR	Isolation	
	Results	Reactive serovar	Final title		Kidney	Urine
01	Negative	-	-	Negative	Negative	Negative
02	Negative	-	-	Negative	Negative	Negative
03	Positive	Butembo	100	Positive	Negative	Negative
04	Negative	-	-	Negative	Negative	Negative
05	Positive	Butembo	100	Positive	Negative	Negative
06	Negative	-	-	Negative	Negative	Negative
07	Positive	Butembo	100	Negative	Negative	Negative
08	Negative	-	-	Negative	Negative	Negative
09	Positive	Butembo	100	Positive	Negative	Negative
10	Positive	Butembo	200	Negative	Negative	Negative
11	Positive	Butembo	100	Negative	Negative	Negative
12	Negative	-	-	Negative	Negative	Negative
13	Negative	-	-	Negative	Negative	Negative
14	Positive	Butembo	100	Negative	Negative	Negative
15	Negative	-	-	Negative	Negative	Negative
16	Negative	-	-	Negative	Negative	Negative
17	Positive	Butembo	100	Negative	Negative	Negative
18	Negative	-	-	Negative	Negative	Negative
19	Negative	-	-	Negative	Negative	Negative
20	Positive	Butembo	100	Negative	Negative	Negative
Total	9	Butembo	100, 200	3	0	0

Table 6. Demonstration of the diagnosis of Ieptospirosis in the biological samples analyzed, belonging to herd 6 and coming from the municipality of Ponta de Pedras, according to the technique used, Belém, 2007.

Sample	SAM			MAR-	Isolation	
	Results	Reactive serovar	Final title		Kidney	Urine
01	Positive	Butembo	400	Positive	Positive	Negative
02	Negative	-	-	Positive	Negative	Negative
03	Negative	-	-	Positive	Negative	Negative
04	Negative	-	-	Negative	Negative	Negative

05	Negative	-	-	Positive	Negative	Negative
06	Negative	-		Negative	Negative	Negative
07	Positive	Autumnalis	100	Negative	Negative	Negative
08	Negative	-		Negative	Negative	Negative
09	Negative	-	-	Negative	Negative	Negative
10	Positive	Butembo	100	Positive	Positive	Negative
11	Negative	-	-	Negative	Negative	Negative
12	Positive	Butembo	100	Negative	Negative	Negative
13	Positive	Butembo	200	Positive	Negative	Negative
14	Positive	Butembo	100	Positive	Negative	Negative
15	Positive	Butembo	100	Positive	Negative	Negative
16	Positive	Butembo	100	Negative	Negative	Negative
17	Positive	Butembo	100	Positive	Negative	Negative
18	Negative	-	-	Negative	Negative	Negative
19	Positive	Butembo	100	Negative	Negative	Negative
20	Positive	Butembo	200	Negative	Negative	Negative
Total	11	Autumnalis Butembo	100, 200, 400	9	2	0

Table 7. Demonstration of the diagnosis of leptospirosis in the biological samples analyzed, belonging to herd 7 and coming from the municipality of Salvaterra, according to the technique used, Belém, 2007.

Sample	SAM			MAR	Isolation	
	Results	Reactive serovar	Final title		Kidney	Urine
01	Positive	Hardj o	100	Positive	Positive	Positive
02	Negative	-	-	Negative	Negative	Negative
03	Positive	Butembo	200	Positive	Negative	Negative
04	Positive	Hardj o	200	Positive	Negative	Negative
05	Positive	Butembo	200	Negative	Negative	Negative
06	Positive	Hardj o	100	Positive	Negative	Negative
07	Positive	Hardj o	200	Negative	Negative	Negative
08	Negative	-	-	Negative	Negative	Negative
09	Positive	Hardj o	200	Negative	Negative	Negative
10	Negative	-	-	Negative	Negative	Negative

11	Positive	Butembo	100	Negative	Negative	Negative
12	Positive	Hardj o	200	Negative	Negative	Negative
13	Positive	Pomona	200	Positive	Negative	Negative
14	Negative	-	-	Negative	Negative	Negative
15	Negative	-	-	Negative	Negative	Negative
16	Positive	Hardj o	200	Positive	Negative	Negative
17	Positive	Hardj o	400	Positive	Negative	Negative
18	Positive	Butembo	200	Positive	Negative	Negative
19	Positive	Hardj o	200	Positive	Negative	Negative
20	Positive	Butembo	100	Positive	Positive	Negative
Total	15	Butembo Hardj o Pomona	100, 200, 400	10	2	1

Table 8. Demonstration of the diagnosis of Ieptospirosis in the biological samples analyzed, belonging to herd 8 and coming from the municipality of Muanà, according to the technique used, Belém, 2007.

Sample	SAM			MAR-	Isolation	
	Results	Reactive serovar	Final title		Kidney	Urine
01	Positive	Castellonis	200	Negative	Negative	Negative
02	Positive	Hardj o	100	Negative	Negative	Negative
03	Positive	Hardj o	100	Negative	Negative	Negative
04	Negative	-	-	Negative	Negative	Negative
05	Negative	-	-	Positive	Negative	Negative
06	Negative	-	-	Negative	Negative	Negative
07	Positive	Hardj o	200	Negative	Negative	Negative
08	Positive	Hardj o	100	Negative	Negative	Negative
09	Negative	-	-	Negative	Negative	Negative
10	Positive	Hardj o	200	Negative	Negative	Negative
11	Positive	Hardj o	200	Negative	Negative	Negative
12	Negative	-	-	Negative	Negative	Negative
13	Positive	Pomona	200	Negative	Negative	Negative
14	Negative	-	-	Negative	Negative	Negative
15	Positive	Castellonis	200	Negative	Negative	Negative

16	Positive	Hardj o	100	Negative	Negative	Negative
17	Negative	-	-	Positive	Negative	Negative
18	Positive	Bratislava	100	Negative	Negative	Negative
19	Positive	-	-	Negative	Negative	Negative
20	Positive	Hardj o	100	Positive	Negative	Negative
Total	12	Bratislava Castellonis Pomona	Hardjo, 100, 200	3	0	0

Table 9. Demonstration of the diagnosis of leptospirosis in the biological samples analyzed, belonging to herd 9 and coming from the municipality of Chaves, according to the technique used, Belém, 2007.

Sample	SAM			MAR	Isolation	
	Results	Reactive serovar	Final title		Kidney	Urine
01	Positive	Hardj o	200	Positive	Negative	Negative
02	Positive	Hardj o	200	Negative	Negative	Negative
03	Negative	-	-	Negative	Negative	Negative
04	Negative	-	-	Negative	Negative	Negative
05	Negative	-	-	Positive	Negative	Negative
06	Positive	Autumnalis	200	Negative	Negative	Negative
07	Positive	Hardj o	200	Positive	Negative	Negative
08	Negative	-	-	Positive	Negative	Negative
09	Negative	-	-	Negative	Negative	Negative
10	Positive	Hardj o	200	Negative	Negative	Negative
11	Positive	Hardj o	100	Negative	Negative	Negative
12	Negative	-	-	Negative	Negative	Negative
13	Negative	-	-	Negative	Negative	Negative
14	Negative	-	-	Negative	Negative	Negative
15	Negative	-	-	Positive	Negative	Negative
16	Positive	Autumnalis	200	Positive	Negative	Negative
17	Negative	-	-	Negative	Negative	Negative
18	Positive	Hardj o	200	Negative	Negative	Negative
19	Negative	-	-	Negative	Negative	Negative
20	Negative	-	-	Negative	Negative	Negative

Total	8	Autumnalis Hardj o	100, 200	6	0	0

Table 10. Demonstration of the diagnosis of leptospirosis in the biological samples analyzed, belonging to herd 10 and coming from the municipality of Cachoeira do Arari, according to the technique used, Belém, 2007.

Sample	SAM			- MAR -	Isolation	
	Results	Reactive serovar	Final title		Kidney	Urine
01	Positive	Butembo	100	Negative	Negative	Negative
02	Negative	-	-	Negative	Negative	Negative
03	Negative	-	-	Negative	Negative	Negative
04	Negative	-	-	Negative	Negative	Negative
05	Negative	-	-	Negative	Negative	Negative
06	Negative	-	-	Negative	Negative	Negative
07	Negative	-	-	Negative	Negative	Negative
08	Positive	Hardj o	100	Negative	Negative	Negative
09	Negative	-	-	Negative	Negative	Negative
10	Negative	-	-	Positive	Negative	Negative
11	Negative	-	-	Negative	Negative	Negative
12	Positive	Hardj o	100	Negative	Negative	Negative
13	Negative	-	-	Positive	Negative	Negative
14	Negative	-	-	Negative	Negative	Negative
15	Negative	-	-	Positive	Negative	Negative
16	Negative	-	-	Positive	Negative	Negative
17	Positive	Butembo	100	Positive	Negative	Negative
18	Positive	Butembo	100	Positive	Negative	Negative
19	Positive	Hardj o	100	Positive	Negative	Negative
20	Negative	-	-	Negative	Negative	Negative
Total	6	Butembo Hardj o	100	7	0	0

Of the 200 samples analyzed using SAM, 106 were positive for at least one serovar of *Leptospira spp*, which represents 53% of positivity, while 94 samples did not react to any of the serovars tested, representing 47% of the total. The number of positive samples ranged from six to 15 in the herds, and the percentage of positive samples ranged from 30 to 75% (Table 11).

The descending order of reactive serovars according to the number of positive samples was: Butembo, Hardjo, Autumnalis, Pomona, Castellonis and Pyrogenes, Bratislava and Shermani (Figure 4). The serovars that did not react in any of the samples analyzed were: Australis, Bataviae, Canicola, Whitcombi, Sensot, Hebdomadis, Icterohaemorrhagiae, Copenhageni, Cynopteri, Wolffi, Javanica, Mini, Tarassovi, Panamà, Grippotyphosa, Andamana and Patoc. The number of samples positive for the reactive serovars considering the final titration are shown in Tables 11 and 12 and Figure 05.

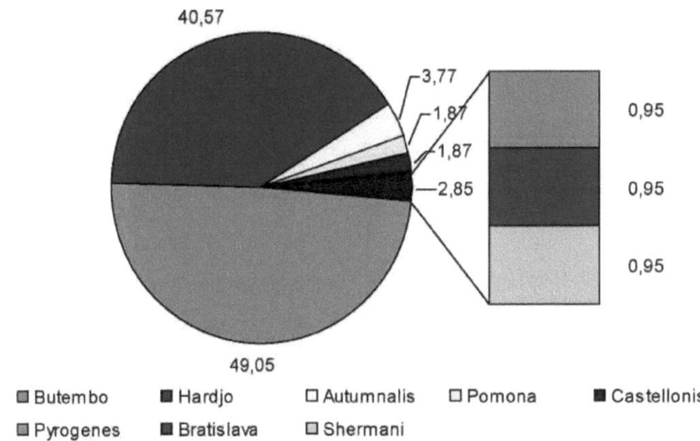

Figure 4 - Representation of the percentage of positivity to reactive serovars, using SAM, Belém, 2007.

Table 11. Demonstration of the number of samples and the percentage of positives to the reactive serovars and the final titration, by SAM, in the herds analyzed, Belém, 2007.

Flocks	Reactive serovars	Titration			Number of positive samples	Total	
		100	200	400		Positive samples	% positive
	Butembo	8	0	1	9		
1						11	55
	Hardjo	2	0	0	2		
	Butembo	2	2	0	4		
	Hardjo	4	0	0	4		
2						10	50
	Pyrogenes	1	0	0	1		
	Shermani	1	0	0	1		
	Butembo	6	2	0	8		

Flocks	Reactive serovars	Titration 100	200	400	Number of positive samples	Total Positive samples	% positive
3						9	45
	Autumnalis	1	0	0	1		
	Butembo	4	0	0	4		
4						15	75
	Hardjo	11	0	0	11		
5	Butembo	8	1	0	9	9	45
	Butembo	7	2	1	10		
6						11	55
	Autumnalis	1	0	0	1		
	Hardjo	2	6	1	9		
7	Butembo	2	3	0	5	15	75
	Pomona	0	1	0	1		
	Hardjo	5	3	0	8		
	Castellonis	0	2	0	2		
8						12	60
	Pomona	0	1	0	1		
	Bratislava	1	0	0	1		
	Hardjo	1	5	0	6		
9						8	40
	Autumnalis	0	2	0	2		
10	Butembo	3	0	0	3	6	30
	Hardjo	3	0	0	3		
Total	-	73	30	3	106	106	53

Figure 05. Representation of the number of reactions found for each reagent serovar, according to the final titration, Belém, 2007.

The final titration of 100 was found in all the herds and was present in 73 positive samples, which represents 68.87% of the reactions. For this titration, there was a range of 1 to 15 reactions in the herds analyzed. As for the sex of the animals, we found 34 reactions in females and 39 in males. At the final titration of 200, 7 herds reacted (except herds 1, 4 and 10), ranging from one to 10 reactions per herd, making up 30 reactions, corresponding to 28.30% of the 106 reactions found. According to gender, there were 12 reactions in males and 18 in females. The final titer of 400 was only found in three samples, belonging to herds 1, 6 and 7, reacting in only one sample from each herd, corresponding to 2.83% of the reactions found. Only the Butembo and Hardjo serovars reacted to this titre, and two samples were from females and one from a male. No sample tested reacted to the titers of 800, 1,600, 3,200 and 6,400.

Table 12. Number of samples and percentage of positives (%), using SAM, according to reactive serovars in the herds analyzed, Belém, 2007.

Sorovar	Reactive flocks	% of groups reagents	No. of samples with final titration			No. of reagents	%
			100	200	400		
Butembo	1, 2, 3, 4, 5 6, 7, 10	80	40	10	2	52	49,05
Hardjo	1, 2, 4, 7, 8, 9, 10	70	28	14	1	43	40,57
Autumnalis	3, 6, 9	30	2	2	0	4	3,77
Pomona	7, 8	20	0	2	0	2	1,87
Castellonis	8	10	0	2	0	2	1,87
Pyrogenes	2	10	1	0	0	1	0,95
Bratislava	8	10	1	0	0	1	0,95
Shermani	2	10	1	0	0	1	0,95
Total	All	-	73	30	3	106	100

The Butembo serovar was the most reactive of all, showing positivity in 52 samples, making up 49.05% of positives. Of all the herds analyzed, only herds 8 and 9 showed no reaction to this serovar. Considering the final titer found, the Butembo serovar reacted to the titer of 100 in 40 of them, and for the titer of 200, this serovar reacted in 10 samples. For the 400 titer, only two samples reacted.

The Hardjo serovar was the second most reactive, showing positive reactions in 43 samples, corresponding to 40.57%. However, it was present in 70% of the herds analyzed. The final titer was 100 in 28 samples. For the 200 titre, the Hardjo serovar reacted in 14 samples, with the highest number of positive samples for this titre. However, only one sample reacted to the 400 titration.

The Autumnalis serovar was positive in 4 samples from 3 herds (herds 3, 6 and 9). It reacted to titers 100 and 200 in 2 positive samples for each titration.

The Pomona serovar was positive in 2 samples and was found in flocks 7 and 8, and reacted only to the 200 titer. The Castellonis serovar reacted in 2 samples from flock 8, and was only positive to the 200 titer.

The Pyrogenes, Bratislava and Shermani serovars were reactive in only one sample at a titre of 100 each and belonged to herds 2, 8 and 2, respectively.

The serological data found using SAM, in terms of the sex of the animals, shows that of the 100 samples of males tested, 52 were positive, which corresponds to 52% positivity. Of the 100 buffalo samples, 54 reacted positively to this test, giving a positivity rate of 54%. If we consider the total number of reactive samples (106), we get 49.06% in males and 50.94% in females (Table 13).

Table 13. Demonstration of the number of samples tested, positives and percentage of positives of the samples tested and percentage of positives of the reagents, using SAM, according to the sex of the animals, Belém, 2007.

Sex	No. of samples tested	No. of samples positive	% of samples tested positive	% positive of reagent samples
Male	100	52	52	49,06
Fèmea	100	54	54	50,94
Total	200	106	53	100

According to MAR, of the 200 blood serum samples analyzed, 55 reacted, which corresponds to 27.5%. The number of positive samples ranged from three to ten per herd. In these terms, the percentage of positive animals ranged from 15% (3/20) to 50% (10/20) in these herds (Table 14).

Table 14. Number of samples tested, reagents and percentage of positives, using MAR, in the herds analyzed, Belém, 2007.

Flocks	Number of serological samples analyzed	Number of positive serological samples	Percentage of positives
1	20	05	25
2	20	03	15
3	20	05	25
4	20	04	20
5	20	03	15
6	20	09	45

7	20	10	50

Flocks	Number of serological samples analyzed	Number of positive serological samples	Percentage of positives
8	20	03	15
9	20	06	30
10	20	07	35
Total	200	55	27,5

The percentage of positive animals in males was 27% and in females 28%. If we consider the 55 reactive samples as a total, 49.09% were males and 50.91% females (Table 15).

From the number and percentage of total positive and negative samples for the two serological tests, we can see that of the 106 (53%) SAM-positive samples, 39 (19.50%) also reacted to MAR and 67 (33.50%) did not react. Of the 94 (47%) SAM-negative samples, 16 (8%) reacted to MAR and 78 (39%) did not react to any serological test. Similarly, of the 200 samples analyzed by SAM and MAR, 106 were positive and 94 negative by the first test, and 55 (27.5%) were positive and 145 (72.5%) negative by the second, respectively (Table 16).

Table 15. Number of samples tested and positive, percentage of positive samples tested and percentage of positive reagents, using MAR, according to the sex of the animals, Belém, 2007.

Sex	No. of samples tested	No. of samples positive	% of samples tested positive	% positive of reagent samples
Male	100	27	27	49,09
Female	100	28	28	50,91
Total	200	55	27,5	100

Table 16. Number and percentage of positive and negative samples using the two serological techniques, Belém, 2007.

MAR	SAM				Total	
	Positive	%	Negative	%	Number of Samples	%
Positive	39	19,5	16	8	55	27,5

Negative	67	33,5	78	39	145	72,5
Total	106	53	94	47	200	100

Using the data in Table 16, the following parameters were determined for the MAR technique: Sensitivity: 39/106 = 36.79%; Specificity: 78/94 = 82.97%; False positives: 16/94 = 17.02%; False negatives: 67/106 = 63.20% and MAR/SAM Concordance Rate: (39+78)/200 = 58.50%. Using the Chi Square test, these results were evaluated and showed a probability of 0.0009 and a significance level of 10.96.

The number of positive and negative samples for the two serological tests was also checked in each herd analyzed. The agreement between the number of positive samples and the two serological tests ranged from 1 to 10 samples, corresponding to 5 to 50%. The number of negative samples varied from 5 to 11, corresponding to 25% to 55% (Table 17).

Table 17. Number of positive samples (P) and percentage of positives (%), using SAM and MAR, in the herds analyzed, Belém, 2007.

Flocks	Number of positive samples				Number of negative samples			
	SAM	MAR	Both	%	SAM	MAR	Both	%
1	11	05	4	20	9	15	8	40
2	10	03	2	10	10	17	9	45
3	9	05	3	15	11	15	9	45
4	15	04	4	20	5	16	5	25
5	9	03	3	15	11	17	11	55
6	11	09	6	30	9	14	6	30
7	15	10	10	50	5	10	5	25
8	12	03	1	5	8	17	6	30
9	8	06	3	15	12	14	9	45
10	6	07	3	15	14	13	10	50
Total	106	55	39	19,5	94	145	78	39

The isolation of *Leptospira spp.* in culture media from kidney and urine samples in the herds analyzed was demonstrated in 13 Marajoara bubalinos. Of the 50 kidney samples analyzed, 12 showed positive growth of the bacteria. Of the 50 urinary samples analyzed, only 3 were positive. The herds that showed the presence of leptospira in the kidneys were 1, 2, 3, 4, 6 and 7. Urine samples with positive leptospira growth were present in herds 2 and 7, and these were the only herds that showed positivity in both urine and kidney. Flocks 5, 8, 9 and 10 showed no leptospira growth in any kidney or urine sample (Table 18).

Table 18. Number of samples analyzed and number of positive samples, by leptospira isolation, in kidney and urine samples, in the herds analyzed, Belém, 2007.

Flocks	Kidney		Urine	
	No. of samples analyzed	sNo. of samples positive	No. of analyzed	samples No. of positive samples
1	5	1	5	0
2	5	3	5	2
3	5	3	5	0
4	5	1	5	0
5	5	0	5	0
6	5	2	5	0
7	5	2	5	1
8	5	0	5	0
9	5	0	5	0
10	5	0	5	0
Total	50	12	50	3

As for the percentage of positivity, 15% of the 100 kidney and urine samples analyzed were positive. However, 24% of these were kidney samples and 6% urine samples. If we analyze the percentage of positives, considering the number of positive samples (15), 80% were renal and 20% urinary (Table 19).

Table 19. Demonstration of the number of samples analyzed, positive, percentage of positive samples tested and percentage of positive total reagents, by leptospira isolation, in total kidney and urine samples, Belém, 2007.

Sample	Number of samples analyzed	Number of positive samples	Percentage of positive test results	Positive percentage of total reagents
Kidney	50	12	24	80

Urine	50	03	6	20
Total	100	15	15	100

As for the sex of the animals, of the 12 positive samples found in the kidney, six were from males and six from females. However, the three positive urine samples all came from females. Overall, of the 15 isolation-positive samples, nine came from females and six from males (Table 20).

The kidney and urine samples positive for the isolation of the agent reacted serologically to only one of these three serovars: Butembo, Hardjo and Autumnalis. The Butembo serovar was reactive in the positive kidney samples from herds 2, 3, 6 and 7, with two positive samples in herds 3 and 6. In herds 2 and 7, only one positive kidney sample also reacted to Butembo. As for the isolation-positive samples that also reacted to Hardjo, we also noticed their presence in four herds: 1, 2, 4 and 7. Herd 2 had two positive kidney samples that reacted to Hardjo, as well as two urine samples. Herd 7 had one positive urine sample (Table 21).

Table 20. Number of samples analyzed (N), positive (P) and percentage (%), by leptospira isolation, according to the sex of the animals, Belém, 2007.

Sex _	Kidney			Urine		
	N	P	%	N	P	%
Male	25	6	24	25	0	0
Female	25	6	24	25	3	12
Total	50	12	24	50	3	6

Table 21. Correlation of the number of positive kidney and urine samples, by leptospira isolation, with the reactive serovars found by SAM, Belém, 2007.

Flocks	No. of positive kidney samples			No. of positive urine samples
	Sorovars			
	Butembo	Hardjo	Autumnalis	Hardjo
1	-	1	-	-
2	1	2	-	2
3	2	-	1	-
4	-	1	-	-

5	-	-	-	-
6	2	-	-	-
7	1	1	-	1
8	-	-	-	-
9	-	-	-	-
10	-	-	-	-
Total	6	5	1	3

Of the 15 serological reactions found, eight were reactive to the Hardjo serovar (five in kidneys and three in urine), which represents 53.33% of the positive samples. The Butembo serovar was reactive in six positive kidney samples (40%) and no urine samples. The Autumnalis serovar was positive in only one sample by isolation and represents 6.67% of the positive samples (Table 22).

Table 22. Demonstration of the percentage of positivity of the correlation between the number of positive kidney and urine samples through the isolation of leptospires, with the reactive serovar, by SAM, Belém, 2007.

Sorovar	No. of positive samples		Total	%
	Kidney	Urine		
Hardjo	5	3	8	53,33
Butembo	6	0	6	40
Autumnalis	1	0	1	6,67
Total	12	3	15	100

Table 23 shows all the information on the samples that were positive, both in kidney and urine, correlating positivity by SAM and MAR.

The positive female samples, both kidney and urine, belong to herds 1, 2 and 7. However, the positive male samples came from herds 3, 4 and 6. In herd 1, only one sample was positive for kidney isolation, reacting to the Hardjo serovar with a maximum titer of 100. This sample did not react to MAR. In herd 2, none of the isolation-positive samples tested positive for MAR. Sample 01 was positive only in the kidney, and reacted to the Hardjo serovar with a final titer of 100. Sample 05 reacted to urine and was positive for Hardjo with a maximum titre of 100. Sample 10 was positive in kidney and reacted to Butembo with a maximum titre of 100. Sample 15 showed isolation in kidney and urine samples and reacted to Hardjo at a maximum titer of 100.

Table 23. Correlation between leptospira isolation-positive samples and serological results (SAM and MAR), considering herd, sex, serovar and final titration, Belém, 2007.

Flock	SAM Sex	Sorovar	Title	- MAR	Isolation	
					Kidney	Urine
1	F	Hardj o	100	Negative	Positive	Negative
2	F	Hardj o	100	Negative	Positive	Negative
	F	Hardj o	100	Negative	Negative	Positive
	F	Butembo	100	Negative	Positive	Negative
	F	Hardj o	100	Negative	Positive	Positive
3	M	Autumnalis	100	Positive	Positive	Negative
	M	Butembo	100	Positive	Positive	Negative
	M	Butembo	100	Negative	Positive	Negative
4	M	Hardj o	100	Negative	Positive	Negative
6	M	Butembo	400	Positive	Positive	Negative
	M	Butembo	100	Positive	Positive	Negative
7	F	Hardj o	100	Positive	Positive	Positive
	F	Butembo	100	Positive	Positive	Negative

In herd 3, one sample was positive in the kidney and reacted to Autumnalis with a maximum titer of 100. This sample proved to be reactive to MAR. Two other samples were positive in the kidney and reacted to the Butembo serovar with a maximum titer of 100, however, only the first one reacted to MAR. In herd 4, one sample was positive in the kidney and reacted to Hardjo at a maximum titer of 100, but did not react to MAR. In herd 6, the isolation-positive samples reacted to MAR, and one sample was positive in the kidney and reacted to Butembo with a final titer of 400. The other sample was also positive in the kidney and reacted to Butembo with a maximum titre of 100. In flock 7, the isolation-positive samples also reacted to MAR and SAM with a final titer of 100. One sample was positive in both kidney and urine and reacted to Hardjo. The other sample was positive only in the kidney and reacted to the Butembo serovar.

The percentage of positives found by isolating leptospires in kidneys, according to the serovar that reacted, is shown in Table 24. Butembo was reactive in 50%, followed by Hardjo with 41.67% and

Autumnalis with 9.10% of the positive kidney samples, and both Hardjo and Butembo showed a percentage of positives of 45.45% for the final titration of 100. Autumnalis only reacted to the final titre of 100, with a positive percentage of 9.10%. None of the isolation-positive samples reacted to a titre of 200. The Butembo serovar was the only one to react at 400 (only one sample).

The direct demonstration of *Leptospira spp* in kidney and urine samples, using PCR, was not positive in any of the samples analyzed.

Table 24. Correlation of the number of samples and the positive serological percentage with the kidney samples positive for leptospira isolation, according to the final titration found, Belém, 2007.

Sorovar	Kidney						Total	
	100	%	200	%	400	%	N	%
Butembo	5	45,45	0	0	1	100	6	50
Hardj o	5	45,45	0	0	0	0	5	41,67
Autumnalis	1	9,10	0	0	0	0	1	8,33
Total 3	11	100	0	0	1	0	12	100

5. Discussion

Difficulties in diagnosing leptospirosis have been the biggest obstacle to understanding many aspects of the disease in cattle herds. For this reason, according to international conventions, the diagnosis of bovine leptospirosis (definitive confirmation of infection) is based on direct and/or indirect testing for leptospires in the animal (Ellis & McDowell, 1993). Based on these parameters, all the herds analyzed had the disease, as demonstrated by the use of SAM and MAR. As for the direct demonstration of the bacteria by isolating the agent in the kidney or urine, 60% of the herds analyzed showed the presence of leptospira in one or more animals.

Although the buffalo species prefers flooded areas, which would lead one to believe that they are resistant to leptospirosis, this is not what was observed in this study or in other serological studies carried out by Brazilian and foreign researchers. Using the SAM test, the serological presence was observed in 100% of the herds analyzed and showed a high prevalence of the disease, which is considered a natural infection in Pará's buffalo herds. The variation in the proportion of reactive buffalo per herd was between 30 and 75%. These data are in line with other serological studies carried out in 22 and 36 buffalo herds in Pará, raised in an extensive system in different regions, where positivity was found in 21 and 35 of them. The variation in the proportion of reactors ranged from 25 to 84.61% in the first study and 25 to 96.87% in the second (Negrao *et al.,* 2002; Negrao *et al.,* 2003).

Serological data has also been observed in cattle in the state, such as by Homem (1999), who evaluated 67 properties in the municipality of Uruarà, and found 97% of them had at least one positive animal, and by Negrao (1999), who found reactor animals in all 23 herds tested. Another high occurrence of the disease in the Amazon region was observed by Aguiar *et al.* (2006), with 95.3% positivity in the 85 herds analyzed in the municipality of Monte Negro, in Rondônia.

The serological results obtained by SAM show that 53% (106/200) of the animals examined had antibodies against at least one serovar of *Leptospira spp.* Similar results were found in other serological studies in Parà, with a seroprevalence of 58.33% (693/1188) in buffalo from herds with and without a history of reproductive disorders (Negrao *et al.,* 2003).

In other Brazilian states, Aguiar, *et al.* (2006), in Rondônia, found a prevalence of 52.8% of positive cows. In Maranhao, the prevalence found was 56.75% (Pereira, *et al.,* 1999), and in Piaui, it was 52.88% of the animals, but all 16 herds analyzed were reactive (Mineiro, 2003). In Sao Paulo, 60.43% of reactors were found in 2,449 cattle from 56 properties in the states of Sao Paulo, Minas Gerais, Rio de Janeiro, Paranà, Rio Grande do Sul and Mato Grosso do Sul (Vasconcellos *et al.*, 1997).

The data found in this study was higher than the prevalence in buffaloes found in Parà, of 38.26% (132/345) of positive animals (Negrao *et al.,* 2001), and 45.49% (369/811) of animals that had abortions and repeated oestrus (Negrao *et al.,* 2003). They were also higher than the serological data in cattle found by Lins *et al.* (1986), who evaluated the occurrence of anti-leptospiral agglutinins and obtained a seroprevalence of 9.3% (5/54) and by Negrao *et al.* (2001), who observed 40.36% (134/332) positivity.

Other lower occurrences were observed in serological surveys of buffaloes carried out in northeastern Brazil, which showed a prevalence of 44.93% (293/652) in Bahia (Dória *et al.,* 1979). In Pernambuco, Oliveira *et al.* (2001) found a 47.83% positive rate when they examined 464 cattle from 15 properties.

In older serological studies carried out at the Sao Paulo Biological Institute between 1974 and 1980, Giorgi *et al.* (1981) found 6.71% (57/849) of positive buffaloes and 15.5% (2,736/17,643) of cattle. More recently, in a retrospective serological survey carried out between 1984 and 1997, Fâvero *et al.* (2002) examined 879 buffaloes and found seropositivity in 43.7% of these animals. Also in Sao Paulo, 37.7% (152/403) were found in buffaloes in the Ribeira Valley and 45.56% (1258/2761) in cattle in the municipality of Botucatu (Langoni *et al.,* 1997; Langoni *et al.,* 2000).

In Mato Grosso do Sul, buffalo living in the wild were analyzed and found to be 41% (16/39) positive (Girio *et al.,* 2004). In Paranà, Rodrigues *et al.* (1999) surveyed 1253 female cattle from 14 dairy farms and found 13.25% of positive animals on 10 farms.

Other lower occurrences in buffalo were found in India (two studies) and Pakistan, with 10%, 35.1% and 33% positivity, in 47, 57 and 932 samples, respectively (Upadhye *et al.,* 1981; Ratnam *et al.,* 1994; Chaudhry *et al.*, 1996).

The data found in this study were lower than those of Molnar *et al.* (1995), who found a seroprevalence in buffalo of 96.7% (32/33), and Molnar *et al.* (2000), who analyzed 131 cattle from seven herds in Pará, and found a seropositivity proportion of 74.7% of reactors. In another study, 65.9% (275/417) of cattle slaughtered in a slaughterhouse for human consumption were reactive (Negrao, 1999). In another serological survey carried out in Parà, on buffaloes destined for slaughter, the seroprevalence was 85.94% (324/377) of positive animals (Negrao *et al.,* 2003).

In Bahia, Caldas *et al.* (1997) found 82.8% (116/120) of reactive cattle. In the state of Goiás, the prevalence of leptospirosis in dairy cattle was estimated at 81.90% of reactive animals in 20 properties sampled in the Goiânia micro-region (Juliano *et al.,* 2000). In Italy, a prevalence of 67% (293/437) was detected, ranging from 42 to 100% in the buffalo herds studied (Ciceroni *et al.,* 1995).

The positivity of all the herds, taking into account their variations, as well as the high prevalence in the Marajoara bubal population analyzed, is due to the dynamics of the epidemiology of leptospirosis, caused by environmental conditions or health management that favors it. The main factor is the environmental conditions of the Amazon region. Although its waters are acidic, this is not a limiting factor, but the pH of the soil (neutral to alkaline), high rainfall, high relative humidity and ambient temperature, as well as the presence of free-living wild animals cohabiting with bubalinos, favor the permanence of leptospira in the wild and the development of the disease in susceptible animals (Faine, 1982; Lins, 1982; Homem, 1999).

Another aspect that should be considered is the health status of the Marajoara herds, since the vast majority of them have poor health management conditions (Moura Carvalho *et al.,* 2002). Factors that make it possible for the disease to spread are the entry of animals into the properties from others with unknown health conditions, breeding without criteria for separating the animals by sex and age, and the cohabitation of pubescent and impubescent animals (Genovez, 1999; Ellis, 1994). Rural properties located in regions with these environmental conditions and which also do not adopt vaccination programs against Ieptospirosis, nor the practice of periodic examinations of animals destined for reproduction, will probably have a high prevalence and consequently high rates of reproductive problems (Miller, *et al.,* 1991; Vasconcellos, *et al.,* 1997).

As for positivity according to the sex of the animals, no significant difference was found, since of the 106 serologically reactive samples, 50.94% (54/106) were from females and 49.06% (52/106) from males. These data are in line with what the literature has stated that leptospirosis has no predilection for sex (Ellis & McDowell, 1993; Ellis, 1994).

Similar data was found in Brazil by Abuchaim & Dutra (1985) and Ribeiro *et al.* (1988), who found no relationship between serological prevalence and the sex of the animals studied. Similarly, Miller *et al.* (1991) found a seroprevalence of 55% in females and 45% in males when they analyzed cattle destined for slaughter in Puerto Rico. Girio & Mathias (1989) also found no significant differences between females (19.05%) and males (15.45%) when analyzing dairy herds. The only divergent finding was that of Langoni *et al.* (2000), who found that females had a higher number of reactors than males, with 47.57% and 1.25% of reactors, respectively.

Most of the leptospirosis surveys carried out in Brazil have been aimed at the female population, because dairy farms are the ones that show the most clinical signs of the disease and/or have low reproductive indices (Girio *et al.,* 1990; Santana et *al.,* 1997; Rodrigues *et al.,* 1999; Juliano *et al.,* 2000). However, Brod *et al.* (1995) serologically compared dairy and beef herds with reproductive disorders and found a higher prevalence for beef herds, with 71.80% compared to 42.62% for dairy herds.

The serological results of this study showed the highest number of reactions for a titre of 100 (73 samples), but there were reactions for 200 (30 samples) and 400 (3 samples). Knowing that titres above 100 are consistent with infection, the other titres found determine the serological results in a population of animals with greater certainty, which should be considered by the final titre of the most reactive serovar within a population (Vasconcellos *et al.,* 1997). For the diagnosis of leptospirosis in humans or in other animal species where it is important to confirm the individual diagnosis, there is a need for paired serology to assess the increase or decrease in antibody titres (Ellis & McDowell, 1993).

The seroprevalence of the serovars analyzed was surprising, since Butembo was the most reactive with 49.05% (52/106), and was the most widespread in the herds analyzed, being present in 80% of them. It titrated 100 in 40 samples, 200 in 10 samples and 400 in two samples. Although most of the positive samples only reacted to the 100 titre, the other samples that reacted to the 200 and 400 titres are extremely important in the epidemiological demonstration of Butembo in buffaloes in the state of Parâ.

These data show a regional serological reality, as they are confirmed in the state of Parà, by serology carried out on buffaloes that proved to be reactive in

32.75% (227/693) of slaughter animals from 14 herds, with titers between 200 and 400, although, in another population of animals, they showed reactions in only three properties with reproductive disorders (Negrao *et al.,* 2003).

In a survey of 22 buffalo herds in the state, 7.58% of the buffaloes reacted to Butembo, with a maximum titration of 200 (Negrao *et al.,* 2002). In another study of buffaloes and cattle from Pará, the seroprevalence for Butembo in the former was 17.42% (2nd place) and in the latter it was 3.73% (10th place), with a titration of 100 (Negrao *et al.*, 2001). Also in the state of Parà, positive serology for Butembo was found in wild animals, without detailing the percentage of positives (Lins & Lopes, 1984).

Divergent results for Butembo in the state were shown by Homem (1999), who found that 1.5% of the samples were reactive and that they also showed cross-reactions with Pomona, Grippotyphosa and Pyrogenes and only at a titre of 100. In Rondônia, only 0.9% (10/1114) of reactors were detected and they belonged to 9.7% (8/82) of the properties studied (Aguiar *et al.,* 2006).

In other states of the Federation, the only seroprevalence data for Butembo in buffaloes was found in Bahia, with 6.21% (25/401) of positives with titers ranging from 100 to 400 (Dória *et al.,* 1979). In cattle, only one study showed positive animals with titers above 100, in which of 30 reactor animals, 19 were positive at 100, three at 200, two at 400, two at 800 and four at 3,200 (Viegas *et al.,* 1980). In other studies on cattle, only seroprevalence to Butembo with a titer of 100 was found, described in Paranà, which found 7.83% (13/166) of reactors; in Minas Gerais which found 0.5% (82/16923) and in Piaui which found a low prevalence without detailing the percentage of positives (Rodrigues *et al.,* 1999; Mineiro, 2003; Araùjo *et al.,* 2005). In Santa Catarina, 10.4% of dogs tested positive for Butembo (Blazius, *et al.,* 2005).

No other serological study of epidemiological importance in cattle carried out in Brazil showed Butembo with significant results, perhaps because it was not included in the battery of antigens tested, such as the studies by Giorgi *et al.* (1981), Abuchaim & Dutra (1985), Ribeiro *et al.* (1988), Moreira (1994) and Langoni et *al.* (2000), or it was included but did not show any relevant results, such as Brod et al. (1995), Vasconcellos et al. *(*1997), Fàvero *et al.* (2002) and Girio et *al. (*2004).

In other countries, positive serology for Butembo has only been reported in Ethiopia, which showed a predominance of this serovar in horses, cattle, sheep, goats, camels and canines, and in the United States, with positivity in 10% (10/101) of the coyotes analyzed (Moch *et al.,* 1975; Marler *et al.,* 1979).

The Butembo serovar was isolated worldwide from only one human case of leptospirosis, in Zaire, Africa, in 1946. This strain was found serologically to be distinct from other serovars available at the time. However, with the subsequent classification scheme for leptospires, it was not listed as a distinct serovar. Later, this strain was studied by Alexander *et al.* (1959), who described it as a new serovar named Butembo, and suggested placing it in the same group as the Cynopteri serovar, due to their similarities, but it was only classified in this serogroup in 1967. However, Dikken & Kmety's (1978) suggested including it in the Autumnalis serogroup, as they observed that it was more closely related. At the Taxonomy Committee meeting in 1986, this arrangement was approved (University of Belgrade, 1997).

Antibodies against the Hardjo serovar were found in 40.57% (43/106) of the serological samples and in 70% of the herds. It was the second most widespread in the herds analyzed and the second most reactive serovar. It showed titers of 100 in 28 samples, 200 in 14 samples and 400 in only one sample. These final titers of 200 and 400 found are also of paramount importance in the epidemiological role of Hardjo in buffalo in this geographical region, given that this serovar usually reacts with low titers in cattle, as they are adapted hosts (Ellis, 1994). This data is in line with recent observations in the state of Parà, Brazil and other countries, and shows that in recent years, this serovar has been the most frequent in cattle on several continents (Vasconcellos, *et al.,* 1997).

In the state of Parà, the few serological surveys of buffaloes have detected Hardjo as the most reactive and widespread in the population studied, as shown by the following results: 52.84% of reactors in 19 of the 22 herds studied (Negrao *et al.,* 2002), and 31.81% positive and present in all herds (Negrao *et al.,* 2001). High endemicity of Hardjo has also been demonstrated, with titres of up to 400 in the Pará herds surveyed (Negrao *et al.,* 2003). In cattle, the Hardjo serovar also proved to be widespread in the population studied in Pará, with serological data of 21.7%, 20.1% and 29.85% (Moreira, 1982; Negrao, 1999; Negrao *et al.,* 2001). In another study in Uruarà, in 61.2% of the herds, the Hardjo serovar was indicated as the most probable (Homem, 1999). In Amazonas and Rondônia, seroprevalence rates of 30.2% and 14.5% of positives were found (Moreira, 1982; Aguiar *et al.,* 2006).

In other Brazilian states, the only high serological data for Hardjo in buffalo was found in Sao Paulo, with 43.3% of reactors (Fàvero *et al.,* 2002). In Mato Grosso do Sul and Bahia, the prevalence was low, with insignificant diffusion in the herds analyzed (Dória *et al.,* 1979; Girio *et al.,* 2004). International data shows Hardjo's endemicity in buffalo only in Italy, with a prevalence of 37% (Ciceroni *et al.,* 1995). In Pakistan, a seroprevalence of 5.5% of reactors in buffaloes was found (Chaudhry *et al.,* 1996). In South Africa, the prevalence of Hardjo in wild buffalo was 1.7% (Myburgh *et al.,* 1990). In India, no study has shown reactivity to Hardjo in buffalo (Upadhye *et al.,* 1981; Ratnam *et al.,* 1994).

In cattle, the prevalence for Hardjo in Brazil was shown in Rondônia (14.5%), Pernambuco (22%), Piaui (39.46%), Sao Paulo (76.78% and 67.57%), Rio de Janeiro (20.98%), Minas Gerais (19.70%, 36.36% and 52.5%), Paranà (10.84%), Rio Grande do Sul (85.25%) and Goiàs (5.20%) (Aguiar *et al.,* 2006; Oliveira *et al.,* 2001; Mineiro, 2003; Vasconcellos *et al.,* 1997; Langoni et *al.,* 2000; Lilenbaum et al., 1995; Araùjo et al., 2005; Ribeiro et al., 1988; Moreira, 1994; Rodrigues *et al.,* 1999; Brod *et al.,* 1995; Juliano et *al.,* 2000).

In several countries, positive titers for the Hardjo serovar have been found in cattle (Kingscote, 1985; Caballero *et al.,* 1989; Bennett, 1991; Ratnam *et al.,* 1994; Feresu et *al.,* 1996). It was also the most widespread in all herds, in agreement with Ellis (1994) and Dhaliwal *et al.* (1996), who consider it to be the most widespread cause of abortion in herds, with serological evidence worldwide. Abortions caused by it occur more frequently in the 3rd and 4th month of pregnancy, and the antibody titre decreases and can be below 100 (Genovez, 1999). Other factors that determine the variation in antibody titers are the virulence of the strain, the number of infecting bacteria and the time elapsed between infection and the taking of samples. These factors are responsible for the following situations: 98% of cows have static titers at the time of abortion; 80% of cows with positive serology at the time of abortion have infected fetuses and 20% of carrier animals have no detectable antibodies (Ellis *et al.,* 1982; Galego & Galego, 1994).

It is interesting to note that Hardjo is also responsible for other reproductive disorders in cattle, and also in buffalo, such as mastitis, retained placenta and epididymitis, leading to economic losses in breeding (Ellis & McDowell, 1993; Ciceroni *et al.,* 1995).

The third most reactive serovar was Autumnalis, which was positive in 3.77% (4 samples) and was present in 30% of the herds analyzed. It reacted to titers of 100 and 200 in 2 samples each. This serovar belongs, together with Butembo, to the Autumnalis serogroup, and cross-reactions probably occur between them. Butembo should be considered the true reactor, as it had the highest number of positive samples and the highest titers (Faine, 1982).

The data for Autumnalis agrees with the finding of 2.8% of reactive cattle in Rondônia (Aguiar *et al.,* 2006); 3.23% of reactive buffalo in Bahia (Dória *et al.,* 1979) and 0.5% of positive cattle in Minas Gerais (Araùjo *et al.,* 2005). Also in buffaloes, serological tests in Pakistan showed a low prevalence of 4.5% positive (Chaudhry *et al.,* 1996). In India, in a serological study of various species of domestic animals, the highest prevalence of Autumnalis and titers of up to 25,600 were found in goats. A good prevalence was found in buffaloes and cattle, although they were not the most reactive (Ratnam *et al.,* 1994). However, in Italy, no reactive buffaloes were found for this serovar (Ciceroni *et al.,* 1995). In serological studies on cattle from Pará, there were also no reactors (Moreira, 1982; Homem, 1999; Negrao, 1999; Molnàr *et al.,* 2000; Negrao *et al,* 2001).

Discordant data for Autumnalis were found in cattle in Paranà, with 14.46% positive (Rodrigues, *et al.,* 1999) and in buffaloes in Parà, with 10.60% and 15.71% reactors, with antibody titers up to 200 (Negrao et al., 2001; Negrao *et al.*, 2002).

Pomona and Castellonis were the 4th most reactive serovars, with 1.87% (2 samples each), reactive only to the 200 titer, with the former found in 2 herds and the latter in only one. Similar results for Pomona in cattle were found in Pernambuco and Rondônia with 1.3% (Oliveira *et al.,* 2001; Aguiar et *al.,* 2006); in Rio Grande do Sul, with 3.15% (Brod *et al.,* 1995); in Goiàs with 2.30% (Juliano et *al.,* 2000); in Sao Paulo with 3.57% (Vasconcellos *et al.,* 1997) and in Minas Gerais with 2.8% (Araùjo et *al.,* 2005).

In the state of Parà, divergent results were shown in 6.7% of cattle (Moreira, 1982), and in 11.11% of buffalo in five properties out of 22 analyzed (Negrao *et al.,* 2002). In wild buffalo in Mato Grosso do Sul it was the most reactive (Girio *et al.,* 2004). A high prevalence was found in cattle in Paranà, with 21.08% (Rodrigues *et al.,* 1999); 11.80% in the Porto Alegre dairy basin (Abuchaim & Dutra, 1985); 10.81% in Sao Paulo (Langoni *et al.,* 2000) and 7.88% in the Minas Gerais triangle (Ribeiro *et al.,* 1988).

Serological data found for Pomona were also divergent in India, with one study showing it to be the most reactive and another study showing it to be the least reactive (Upadhye *et al.*, 1981; Ratnam *et al.,* 1994). Similarly, Chaudhry *et al.* (1994), in Pakistan, detected a low prevalence of this serovar in buffaloes.

In the 1970s and 1980s, the Pomona serovar proved to be one of the most reactive in the bovine population analyzed, second only to Wolffi (Sandoval *et al.,* 1979; Giorgi *et al.,* 1981; Yasuda *et al.,* 1982). This is due to the fact that the immune response of an animal infected by Pomona is quite intense, usually observed by high antibody titers. This occurs more commonly in accidental infections in cattle all over the world. However, in this study this was not observed (titers up to 200), nor in recent surveys of cattle in Brazil and worldwide, perhaps because there is greater specialization in the breeding of production animals, and this has consequently led to a decrease in direct contact with pigs, which are considered to be its reservoirs (Giorgi *et al,* 1981; Ellis & McDowell, 1993).

The serological results found for Castellonis are similar to other studies which have found a low prevalence in cattle (Brod *et al.,* 1995; Juliano et *al.*, 2000; Aguiar et *al.,* 2006), or even, as in other countries, the absence of reactions in the animals studied (Upadhye et al., 1981; Ratnam et al., 1994; Chaudhry et *al.,* 1996). Our data differ from Langoni *et al.* (2000), who found 4.13% of reactors in cattle in Sao Paulo. Higher results were found in buffaloes in Bahia (8.45%), Pernambuco (7.59%) and Parà (7.04%) (Dòria *et al.,* 1979; Oliveira *et al.,* 2001; Negrao et *al.,* 2002). Langoni *et al.* (1997) found high values for Castellonis in buffalo, without specifying the percentage of positives.

The Castellonis serovar was considered by Langoni *et al.* (1995) to be the second most prevalent in sheep. This suggests that infections are related to the presence of sheep on the property, when large numbers of animals with higher titers are found. In the present study, the prevalence found for Castellonis is probably due to cross-reactions with other serovars, because there are almost no sheep farms near the Marajoara flocks studied.

Serological results for the Bratislava, Pyrogenes and Shermani serovars indicate only one positive sample (0.95%) with a final titration of 100. These data are in line with research carried out on buffaloes and cattle in Pará (Moreira, 1982; Homem, 1999; Negrao, 1999; Molnar *et al.,* 2000; Negrao et al., 2001; Negrao et *al.,* 2003), except for Bratislava (Homem, 1999; Negrao, 1999) (Moreira, 1982; Negrao *et al.,* 2001) which showed higher serological frequencies in cattle. In Rondônia, the prevalence was very low (Aguiar *et al.,* 2006).

Results with a low prevalence of these serovars found in this study are always to be expected when using SAM, since this technique uses a battery of live antigens representing the serogroups that occur most frequently in Brazil. Such use promotes numerous cross-reactions for those serovars with greater antigenic affinities, not least because there were few samples that reacted to these serovars, even with low antibody titers, and in these cases they are not considered important for herd diagnosis (Vasconcellos, 1987).

In buffaloes, the only mention of Bratislava was the finding of 7.85% of reactors in Pará (Negrao *et al.,* 2002) and a very low prevalence in Sao Paulo (Langoni *et al.*, 1997). The Bratislava serovar was the second most reactive in cattle in various regions of Pará, and in humans it was the most common (Homem, 1999; Negrao, 1999) and in Pernambuco and Piaui (Oliveira *et al.,* 2001; Mineiro, 2003). It has also been demonstrated in other Brazilian regions, with 35.1% and 7.1 of reactors in Minas Gerais (Moreira, 1994; Silva *et al.,* 1994), 10.24% in Paranà (Rodrigues *et al.,* 1999) and 9.1% in Rio de Janeiro (Lilenbaum *et al.,* 1995). It has also been described in other species such as dogs, pigs and horses, causing clinical leptospirosis (Brem *et al.,* 1990; Miller *et al.,* 1991). Santana *et al.* (1997) found the Bratislava serovar to be the most reactive in cattle with a history of repeated oestrus.

The Shermani serovar is not frequently found in cattle, and the only reports in the literature are 1.35% in buffalo (Negrao *et al.,* 2002), 3.73% in cattle from Pará (Negrao *et al.,* 2001) and very low prevalence in Piaui and Rondônia (Mineiro, 2003; Aguiar *et al.,* 2006). In other animal species, there have been reports of positive titres in pigs, rodents, goats, sheep and dogs (Santa Rosa, 1970; Ciceroni *et al,* 1997).

The serovars that did not react in any of the samples analyzed were: Australis, Bataviae, Canicola, Whitcombi, Sensot, Hebdomadis, Icterohaemorrhagiae, Copenhageni, Cynopteri, Wolffi, Javanica, Mini, Tarassovi, Panamà, Grippotyphosa, Andamana and Patoc.

In various serological surveys carried out in Brazil and around the world, there are differences in serological data, mainly because some of these serovars, such as Hebdomadis, Icterohaemorrhagiae, Wolffi and Grippotyphosa, cause accidental infection in cattle.

In Parà, 3.78% and 1.89% of reactors to Hebdomadis were found in buffaloes (Negrao *et al,* 2001; Negrao *et al,* 2003). Divergent data was found in 18.20% and 16.41% of reactors in cattle from Pará (Negrao, 1999; Negrao *et al.,* 2001). In no foreign literature has the Hebdomadis serovar been found to react in buffalo. In Brazilian cattle, the prevalence varied, with 1.7% in Minas Gerais (Araùjo *et al.,* 2005), 2.48% in Rio Grande do Sul (Brod *et al.,* 1995), 6.63% in Paranâ (Rodrigues *et al.,* 1999), 12.16% in Piaui (Mineiro, 2003) and 34.1% of reactors in Rondônia (Aguiar *et al.,* 2006).

Data found for the Icterohaemorrhagiae serovar were 4.54% and 2.71% of reactive buffaloes in Pará (Negrao *et al,* 2001; Negrao et al, 2002), and also low prevalence in Sao Paulo (Yasuda et al., 1982; Langoni *et al.,* 1997). Quite different findings were found in Bahia, with 0.99% of positives, in Pakistan, which found the Icterohaemorrhagiae serovar to be the most reactive, present in 22.6%

of positive buffalo, and in Kenya in 15.5% of wild buffalo (Dória et al., 1979; Chaudhry et al., 1996; Girio et *al.,* 2004). In Brazil, divergent results have also been demonstrated in cattle from different regions. It was shown to be the most reactive in cows from the Londrina dairy basin, in Paranà, with a prevalence of 28.91% (Rodrigues *et al.,* 1999). Also in a dairy herd in the Goiânia micro-region, it was the second most reactive, with 20.50% of reactors (Juliano *et al.,* 2000). A low frequency was also observed in Minas Gerais, with 0.4% (Araùjo *et al.*, 2005), in Sao Paulo with 3.97% (Langoni *et al.,* 2000), in Rio Grande do Sul, with 0.7% (Abuchaim & Dutra, 1985) and in Piaui and Pernambuco, which did not specify the prevalence (Oliveira *et al.,* 2001, Mineiro, 2003). The total absence of reactors for Icterohaemorrhagiae was observed in the municipality of Uruarà (PA) and in Rondônia (Homem, 1999; Aguiar *et al.,* 2006).

In a retrospective study carried out on various species of domestic animals, it was the most reactive in goats and horses (Fàvero *et al.,* 2002). It also showed high

prevalence in sheep, in 51.25% of them (Langoni *et al.,* 1995) and in goats, in the frequency of 16.87%, being the second most reactive (Alves, *et al.,* 1996).

As rodents are the universal reservoirs of the Icterohaemorrhagiae serovar (Vasconcellos, 1987), it is certain that rodent control must be a very important measure when reactors to it are observed. This is extremely important in outbreaks of human leptospirosis since, in addition to being the most pathogenic to humans, it is more frequent in outbreaks observed in large cities after floods and even in rural areas (Faine, 1982; Corrêa & Corrêa, 1992).

The Grippotyphosa serovar was found in 6.06% and 2.71% of Pará buffaloes (Negrao *et al.,* 2001; Negrao *et al.,* 2002). In Bahia, 4.47% of buffaloes were found to be reactors (Dória *et al.,* 1979). Several studies in São Paulo have shown Grippotyphosa to be one of the most reactive in buffaloes (Giorgi *et al.* 1981; Yasuda et al., 1982; Langoni *et al.,* 1997). International data has only shown it in Pakistan, with 2.6% of positives (Chaudhry *et al.,* 1996).

Previously, this serovar was considered one of the most important in the pathology of the disease in cattle, which showed seroprevalence consistent with infection (Ellis, 1984; Ellis & McDowell, 1993). In Brazilian serological results, positivity was found in 5.6% in Parà (Moreira, 1982), and more recently, 0.2% in Minas Gerais (Araùjo *et al.,* 2005), 0.85% in Pernambuco (Oliveira *et al.,* 2001) and two reactive animals in Rondônia (Aguiar *et al.,* 2006). This serovar has already been isolated from humans in Brazil (Corrêa, 1975) and from wild animals, such as the armadillo *(Dasypus novemcintus)* (Lins & Lopes, 1984), confirming the hypothesis that wild animals in the region act as a reservoir (Homem, 1999).

The Wolffi serovar was found in 6.06% and 12.73 of buffaloes from Pará (Negrao *et al.,* 2001;

Negrao *et al.,* 2002). It proved to be the most reactive in studies conducted in Sao Paulo (Santa Rosa *et al.,* 1970; Girgi *et al.,* 1981; Girio, 1984, Langoni *et al.,* 1997). Fâvero *et al.* (2002) found it to be the second most reactive, with 32.5% of positives. In Bahia, Dória *et al.* (1979) found 46.51% of positive buffalo reactors. No foreign literature has shown reactors to this serovar in buffalo.

In cattle, it was found as the most reactive in 854 positive samples (Giorgi *et al.,* 1981); in 70.59% in Sao Paulo (Langoni et *al.,* 2000), in 40.6% in the Triângulo Mineiro (Ribeiro et *al.,* 1988), in 36.10% of cows in the micro-region of Goiânia (Juliano et *al.,* 2000); in 51.8% and in 83.81% in Bahia (Caldas et al., 1977; Dória *et al.,* 1980). As the second most prevalent, it was seen in Mato Grosso with 30% (Madruga *et al.,* 1980); in herds in Rondônia (Aguiar et *al.,* 2006), Minas Gerais (Araùjo *et al.,* 2005), Piaui (Mineiro, 2003), and Rio de Janeiro (Lilenbaum *et al.,* 1995).

Despite the high prevalence of Wolffi cited in most bovine surveys carried out in Brazil, this was not observed in this study, and the low positivity found is probably due to cross-reactions, especially with Hardjo, since they belong to the same serogroup.

The serological results found by MAR show a prevalence of 27.5% (55/200) of positive samples, with reactors in all the herds analyzed and a range of positivity between 15% (3/20) and 50% (10/20). These data are in line with the finding of 23% of reactive buffalo in Pakistan (Chaudhry *et al.,* 1996), but differ from the frequency found in 48.21% of buffalo in Pará (Negrao *et al., 2002)* and 41.92% of sheep in São Paulo (Langoni *et al.,* 1995).

As for positivity in relation to the sex of the animals, no significant difference was found, since 50.91% (28/55) were females and 49.09% (27/55) were males. No data in the literature has linked positivity to MAR and the sex of the animals. In this study, the serological results found for MAR were in line with the results found for SAM, and are in line with what the literature has stated about the disease not having a predilection for sex (Ellis & McDowell, 1993; Ellis, 1994).

The performance of MAR was evaluated by intrinsic characteristics such as sensitivity and specificity. The results of this test were measured and compared with SAM, which is the standard or reference serological test for the diagnosis of leptospirosis, and has established sensitivity and specificity. Thus, it was possible to evaluate the performance of MAR as a diagnostic test for bubaline leptospirosis, where greater positivity was noted for SAM in 9 of the 10 herds analyzed. This was confirmed by the fact that SAM was positive in 53% of the animals and MAR in only 27.5%.

MAR showed low sensitivity (36.79%), which was determined by the 39 reactor samples (19.5%) of the 106 that had reacted to SAM, and 33.5% (78/106) non-reactors, as well as the demonstration of only 16 animals reacting to MAR, which did not react to SAM. Our result was 63.20% false-negative. Sensitivity is the probability of an infected animal being classified as positive by the test. Low sensitivity tests result in a higher number of false-negative animals (Medronho *et al.,* 2002).

In this study, the highest number of MAR-positive animals was found in samples with a final SAM titre of 100 (25 samples), followed by 11 with a titre of 200 and 3 with a titre of 400. These results differ from those found by Pregnolatto (2001) and Weber *et al.* (1984), who observed a higher correlation of MAR positivity when titers of 400 or more were found in the SAM.

The macroagglutination reaction is considered to be a gene-specific screening test and should have good sensitivity. However, Langoni *et al.* (1995) observed frequent false-negative results and a lower frequency of false-positive results in sheep. However, Pregnolatto (2001) analyzed macroagglutination in human samples positive by SAM, and observed that only 32.2% reacted to MAR when the antibody titers were above 6,400, and in titers between 100 and 400, the technique had difficulty in diagnosing positive patients. Similarly, Weber *et al.* (1984) evaluated 259 pigs by SAM and MAR and found greater positivity to MAR in those samples that showed titers of 400 or higher by SAM.

The low sensitivity found by MAR in the present study disagrees with the findings of Caldas *et al.* (1997), who found 84.48% in 116 bovine samples when they analyzed the Canicola, Pomona, Buenos Aires, Jequitaia and Nazarè serovars using this technique, with better performance for the latter. Other studies that found good sensitivity were Silva (1998), who found good sensitivity in canines, including the Icterohaemorrhagiae, Canicola and Copenhageni serovars as antigenic suspensions, and Weber *et al.* (1984) who found 92.3% sensitivity in slaughtered pigs.

The low sensitivity of MAR may also be due to the antigens used in the technique, which consist of a concentrated suspension of leptospires (*"pool"*) inactivated by formaldehyde (according to the Biomanguinhos - Fiocruz - RJ protocol). This rapid diagnostic method for the disease was developed for human leptospirosis and the leptospira serovars included are probably those most reactive to humans. Another important factor to consider is the high frequency of Butembo and Hardjo serovars found in buffaloes, which probably did not cross-react to the serovars contained in the leptospira *pool.*

The specificity found by MAR was 82.97% and 17.02% false positives. Specificity is the probability that an uninfected animal will have a negative result in the diagnostic test. Tests with low specificity result in a higher number of false positives (Medronho *et al.,* 2002). The specificity found in this study is only below the findings of Silva (1998), who found 94.5% in canines. However, it disagrees with the 45.83% found in cattle (Caldas *et al.,* 1997) and 76.4% found in pigs (Weber *et al.,* 1984).

The frequency of false-positives and false-negatives found in this study is in line with Langoni *et al.* (1995), who found that false-negative results were more frequent than false-positives. The MAR/SAM concordance rate was 58.5% of reactive samples and disagrees with the 77.85% found by Caldas *et al.* (1997), as well as the 26.75% concordance found between the two tests (Negrao *et al.,* 2002).

The results found by the correlation between MAR and SAM determined that this technique did not present the necessary indices for safe results for a serological test, and that, as a screening test, it is expected to perform better in terms of sensitivity. Therefore, the diagnosis of leptospirosis in buffaloes cannot be determined by MAR or replaced by it, not even as a screening test, and SAM is still considered the serological test of choice for buffalo leptospirosis. In these terms, our results are in agreement with Molnar *et al.* (2000), who evaluated and compared SAM with another serological test, the enzyme-linked immunosorbent assay (ELISA), and concluded that, as the former showed greater sensitivity and specificity, it had better diagnostic performance for bovine leptospirosis.

The isolation of leptospires in culture media was demonstrated in 13 Marajoara buffaloes, with 10 animals finding the bacteria only in the kidney, two animals showing it in the kidney and urine, and one animal only in the urine. These results are groundbreaking in Marajoara buffaloes.

Our results found 15 positive kidney and urine samples for the isolation of leptospires and showed a 15% positive rate considering the total samples. Of the 50 kidney samples investigated, 12 were isolated and showed a positive rate of 24%. Analyzing the 50 urine samples, only three were positive and showed a 6% positive rate. If we analyze the number of positive samples, the percentage of kidney positives was 80% and urine positives was 20%. Similar data was found by Langoni *et al.* (1999) in 15 out of 120 fetal kidneys from abortions in a São Paulo cattle herd.

As for the sex of the animals, all the positive urinary samples came from females. In the kidneys, the result was proportional, three in kidney samples and three in urine samples. This fact is inexplicable and is in line with the findings of Ellis *et al.* (1986), who were unable to isolate the bacterium from the kidneys of males, despite having isolated it from the kidneys, epididymis, seminal vesicle and testicle.

Isolation of leptospires in buffalo has only been demonstrated in Brazil by Vasconcellos *et al* (2001), in a urinary sample from a cow on a farm in Vale do Ribeira, Sao Paulo. Other isolates in buffalo were those obtained in a case of jaundice in India (Upadhye *et al.,* 1983), an undisclosed strain with no serological correlation obtained from the milk of a cow with mastitis in Pakistan (Ahmed, 1990) and another strain isolated from the kidney of a buffalo in a slaughterhouse in Italy (Telò *et al.,* 1999).

In the state of Parà, the only report of leptospira isolation was in wild animals, such as rodents *(Proechimys sp),* black-eared opossums *(Didelphis marsupialis),* armadillos *(Dasypus novemcinctus) and* coati *(Nasua nasua),* of the serogroups Hebdomadis, Grippotyphosa, and Cynopteri. They have been shown to be reactive to the serovars Bataviae, Butembo, Canicola, Castellonis, Celledoni, Grippotyphosa, Panama, Icterohaemorrhagiae and Wolffi (Lins & Lopes, 1984).

According to a personal statement by Professor Dr. Silvio Arruda Vasconcellos (USP), the first isolate of leptospira in cattle in Brazil was in 1957, by Freitas from an aborted fetus and typified as Pomona. In 1961, Santa Rosa isolated a strain of Icterohaemorrhagiae, also from an aborted fetus. In 1967, Santa Rosa isolated the Guaiacurus strain from a bovine kidney. In 1970, the same author isolated the Goiano strain, also from kidney.

More recently, Moreira (1994) isolated Georgia and Hardjo strains from cow urine. Soon after, Morais (1994) also found Hardjo in the urine of a cow from a dairy herd with reproductive problems.

Direct demonstration of the agent has also been observed in other animal species. Freitas *et al.* (2004) isolated leptospires in 11 of 14 urine samples from dogs, two in three from cattle and two in 36 samples from pigs in Paranà. In slaughter pigs in Sao Paulo, the bacterium was isolated in a kidney sample from an animal serologically positive for Icterohaemorrhagiae and Autumnalis (Shimabukuro *et al.,* 2003).

Leptospires had been isolated from cattle in other countries since the 1970s. The strains found were grouped into the Hebdomadis serogroup, because at the time the Hardjo serovar was included in this serogroup. Subsequently, the Hardjo serovar became part of the Sejroe serogroup (Ellis, 1994). In all these studies, the vast majority were isolated from the kidneys of slaughterhouse cattle (Orr & Little, 1979; White *et al.,* 1982; Thiermann, 1983; Grégorie *et al.,* 1987; Skilbeck et *al.,* 1988).

There have also been reports of leptospires being isolated in other epidemiological situations, such as the strain isolated from the kidney of a newborn calf in a herd with reproductive problems (Giles *et al.*, 1983). Isolation of the bacteria in the reproductive system of males has also been observed (Ellis *et al.,* 1986), as well as in the reproductive system of females, where leptospira has been isolated from the oviduct, uterus, ovary and vaginal mucosa (Ellis *et al.,* 1986). Cabral *et al.* (2000) isolated leptospires from milk in 11.86% of dairy herd animals.

Our results found greater positivity in kidney samples than in urine samples, in agreement with Ellis & Thiermann (1986) who cultured kidney, uterus and oviduct from non-pregnant cows and found greater positivity in kidneys.

Urine cultures for leptospires were found in only three samples (6%), in line with Bolin *et al.* (1989) who found 8% and Magajevski *et al.* (2005) and Vasconcellos *et al.* (2001) who found only one animal. However, McClintock *et al.* (1993) obtained higher numbers, such as 33.1% (56/169) positive for Hardjo and 3.3% (5/169) for Pomona. The low number of positive urine samples is probably due to the greater opportunities for contamination, and also because the leptospira itself dies more easily in this environment (Ellis *et al.,* 1986). Isolation in culture media has been reported to be difficult due to the small quantity of bacteria (Leonard *et al*., 1992).

Kidney culture proved to be more laborious, although a greater number of isolates were found. This is probably due to the culture method used for seeding, as the inoculum is prepared from the innermost part of the kidney, making contamination more difficult at this stage. Another influencing factor is the large number of leptospires present in the kidney, and at the same time, this organ "protects" them from external action and they remain viable until the inoculum is prepared. The temperature at which the kidneys intended for isolation are packed also acts as a protective factor and enables them to remain viable for longer. This was demonstrated by Skilbeck *et al.* (1988), who found that leptospires remained viable for up to 21 days in kidney samples at a temperature of 4° C. However, at -15°C they were not viable for cultivation.

The culture media used have also proved to be efficient due to the addition of antibiotics, as well as the use of the serial dilution methodology for the cultivation of leptospires (Vasconcellos, 1987). EMJH liquid medium plus antimicrobials is the most widely used culture medium today, as it allows leptospira to grow faster than Flether, although the latter does not allow the culture to be contaminated as much as EMJH without antimicrobials (Cabral *et al.,* 2000; Freitas *et al.,* 2004).

The addition of antimicrobials, especially 5-fluorouracil and nalidixic acid, increases the sensitivity of the technique, as it allows only leptospires to grow, as they are resistant to them, without allowing contamination by other bacteria that compete for nutrients in the culture medium (Vidic *et al.,* 1997; Miraglia *et al.,* 2003; Shimabukuro *et al.,* 2003).

However, many researchers who have tried to isolate leptospires in the urine or organs of animals have been unsuccessful, such as Cunha (2001) who tried it in murines, cattle and humans. The isolation of leptospires from biological material from infected animals and/or asymptomatic carriers has always been described as an extremely difficult and laborious diagnostic technique, since the bacterium is very fragile and dies easily outside the host (Santa Rosa, 1970; Ellis & McDowell, 1993).

All the animals that showed leptospires in their urine and/or kidneys had serological reactions by SAM. The serovars that coincidentally reacted in them were Hardjo (53.33%), Butembo (40%) and Autumnalis (6.67%). Renal isolation was demonstrated in 6 samples (50%) reacting to Butembo, 5 samples reacting to Hardjo (41.67) and 1 sample (8.33%) reacting to Autumnalis. Of these samples, only one showed a final titer of 400 (Butembo serovar), while the rest reacted to a final titer of 100.

The animals that tested positive in urine reacted only to the Hardjo serovar, with final titers of 100, although titers of 200 and 400 have been found for this serovar in animals that tested negative in kidney and/or urine isolation. Normally the Hardjo serovar shows low titers when it comes from carrier animals, as cattle and probably buffaloes act as its reservoirs in the wild (Ellis, 1994; Vasconcellos *et al.,* 2001). Serologically negative animals have also been reported to have positive kidney isolates for Hardjo (Bolin *et al.,* 1989).

The isolation of leptospira in kidney and/or urine in Marajoaras bubalinos is an unprecedented finding in the literature, not least because these animals coincidentally reacted to Butembo or Hardjo. Only one isolate of this serovar has been found to date, in a human case in India. As for Hardjo, it has only been found in cattle in Brazil and worldwide, as mentioned above.

The PCR technique showed no positivity in any of the kidney or urine samples investigated. Similar results were observed by Magajevski *et al.* (2005), who detected leptospires in the kidney, semen and urine of five bulls by isolation, but only one urine sample was positive by PCR. Other studies have shown greater positivity by isolation than by PCR, such as Taylor *et al.* (1997) who compared these two techniques in urine samples and found 27 positive animals by isolation and 17 by PCR. Shimabukuro *et al.* (2003) also compared isolation, PCR and SAM in 131 pigs and found 36.64% by SAM and one kidney sample positive by isolation and PCR.

These data disagree with the findings of Heinemann *et al.* (2000) who detected 80% positivity in the semen of bulls from artificial insemination centers in Sao Paulo, although they recognize the possibility of false-positive reactions, since animals that were negative by isolation and SAM were positive by PCR. They also disagree with Van Eys *et al.* (1989), who compared isolation, SAM and PCR and obtained 38.1%, 47.6% and 61.9% positivity, respectively, and Cortez *et al.* (2006), who detected *Leptospira spp* in 3.2% (4/124) of aborted bovine fetuses. Studies to differentiate pathogenic from saprophytic leptospires were carried out by Parma *et al.* (1997), who developed a PCR technique for this purpose.

In the human diagnosis of leptospirosis, earlier positivity has been observed with PCR than with SAM. Ooteman (2001) demonstrated greater sensitivity with SAM (37.6%) than with PCR (29.6%) in human sera, but highlighted a greater earliness for PCR. Merien *et al.* (1995) also pointed out that PCR had earlier results than SAM when analyzing human sera.

Negative PCR results in this study could be due to various factors, such as the methodology used, the infecting serovar and the stage of the disease. The methodology used may have been flawed at any point during processing. It is known that freezing and thawing samples produces false-negatives, as does not completely eliminating epithelial cells, leukocytes and other substances present in the sample through centrifugation (Lucchesi *et al.,* 2004). PCR can also be inhibited by other substances present in the samples such as hemoglobin, sodium, phosphorus and magnesium (Jones & Bej, 1994). Although Scarcelli *et al.* (2003) applied PCR to the kidney and urine of the capuchin monkey and demonstrated the detection of the agent in autolyzed, frozen or poorly preserved kidney samples.

This technique used DNA extracted from a culture of *Leptospira interrogans* serovar Hardjo, strain Hardjoprajitno, as a positive control. Even so, those samples that were proven to be positive for Hardjo, both by SAM and by isolation, were negative to PCR, perhaps because the strains isolated in this study in the kidney and urine are different from those investigated by PCR.

The length of time the disease has lasted can also influence its diagnosis. As leptospirosis is a chronic disease and the colonization of leptospira in the kidneys occurs in an uncertain manner, just like leptospirosis which is intermittent, the renal carrier state is very difficult to demonstrate, even with techniques with high sensitivity and specificity such as PCR (Van Eys *et al.,* 1989; Mèrien *et al.,* 1992; Parma *et al.,* 1997).

PCR is seen as a promising diagnostic technique, as it has high sensitivity and specificity, as well as being quick to perform. It is capable of detecting 10 bacteria, and during the first ten days of the illness it already shows the bacteria (Brown *et al.,* 1995). Unfortunately, these purposes were not fulfilled in this study, since the aim of evaluating this technique was to complement the direct demonstration of the agent in kidney and urine samples from Marajoara buffaloes, so it does not detract from the diagnostic results observed in the ten herds analyzed.

The epidemiological analysis of leptospirosis in the herds analyzed was clarified by the interpretation of the diagnostic techniques used. Of these techniques, two showed significant results and were extremely important for diagnosing the disease in these herds. One was SAM, which as a herd serology test showed and determined the most frequent and prevalent serovars in the region, with their respective final titers. The other was the isolation of leptospira in the kidney and/or urine, which proved to be extremely important for knowledge of serological variants and direct demonstration of the agent in Marajoara buffalo farms. In this way, the isolation of the bacteria indicates the presence of the disease in the herd.

The epidemiological situation found in these herds was quite varied. Most of them had a very defined health status, such as herds 1, 3, 4, 6, 9 and 10, which reacted to two serovars, even showing leptospires in kidney samples, except for herds 9 and 10. Herd 5 was the only one that reacted to only one serovar and without any positive isolations.

Another situation was found in herds 2, 7 and 8, which reacted to between 3 and 4 serovars per herd, probably demonstrating situations of acute or early-stage disease, due to the large number of cross-reactions observed in the animals tested, as well as the presence of chronic disease, especially in those herds with direct evidence of the agent in kidney and/or urine samples.

The herds from Chaves (herds 1, 2 and 9) showed seroprevalence of 40 to 55%, with Butembo and Hardjo being the most important, the latter being present in all 3 herds. Although they didn't show the highest percentages of seroprevalence, they did show positive isolation, in herds 1 and 2, in 4 and 2 kidney and urine samples, respectively, including both kidney and urine samples in one animal from herd 2.

The herds from the municipality of Cachoeira do Arari, herds 3 and 10, showed seroprevalence of 45% and 30%, respectively, and mainly Butembo. Despite this, they also showed positive kidney isolation in 3 animals.

As for the other 5 herds, with 1 representative in the municipalities of Soure, Santa Cruz do Arari, Ponta de Pedras, Salvaterra and Muanà, there were varied results, with positive serological variation from 45% to 75%, with greater importance for Butembo and isolation of the agent in 4 of these herds. Based on these results, we can conclude that the municipalities of Chaves, Cachoeira do Arari, Soure, Ponta de Pedras and Salvaterra are in a chronic and alarming situation with leptospirosis, since the bacteria present in the kidney has probably spread and will spread to susceptible animals and also to humans in contact with carrier animals.

6. CONCLUSIONS

All the herds analyzed were positive for Ieptospirosis using serological techniques, and in 60% *Leptospira spp* was found in kidney and/or urine samples using the culture isolation technique;

S The seroprevalence of leptospirosis was 53% of the buffaloes analyzed and the variation in prevalence between herds was between 30% and 75%;

s The descending order of reactive serovars was: Butembo with 49.05%, Hardjo with 40.57%, Autumnalis with 3.77%, Pomona and Castellonis with 1.87% each and Bratislava, Pyrogenes and Shermani with 0.95% each;

s The descending order of leptospirosis seroprevalence in the municipalities of the Arari micro-region was: Soure and Salvaterra with 75% each, Muanà with 60%, Chaves and Ponta de Pedras with 55% each and Cachoeira do Arari and Santa Cruz do Arari with 45% reactors each;

s There was no difference in seroprevalence according to the sex of the animals, which showed 50.94% in females and 49.06% in males;

s The presence of *Leptospira spp* was demonstrated in 13 buffaloes from the Arari micro-region, using the isolation technique in culture media from kidney and/or urine samples;

s The animals that tested positive for *Leptospira spp*, using the renal and/or urinary isolation technique, came from herds in the municipalities of Chaves, Cachoeira do Arari, Soure, Ponta de Pedras and Salvaterra;

J Of the 12 animals that tested positive using the kidney isolation technique in culture medium, 6 reacted to Butembo, 5 to Hardjo and 1 to Autumnalis, and the 3 animals that tested positive using the urine isolation technique reacted only to Hardjo;

The MAR serological test did not show good sensitivity for use as a screening test for the diagnosis of leptospirosis in buffaloes from the Arari micro-region, Marajó Archipelago;

J By PCR, no kidney or urine sample analyzed showed the presence of *Leptospira spp* in buffaloes from the Arari micro-region, Marajó Archipelago.

7. BIBLIOGRAPHICAL REFERENCES

ABCB - ASSOCIAÇÃO BRASILEIRA DE CRIADORES DE BÙFALOS (on line). Available at http://www.bufalo.com.br/racas. Accessed on 28/11/2005.

ABUCHAIM, D.M., DUTRA, N.L.F. Prevalence of leptospirosis in cattle in the dairy basin of Porto Alegre - RS. **Arquivos da Faculdade Veterinària da UFRGS, 13**: 5560, 1985.

ADEPARA. AGRICULTURAL DEFENSE AGENCY OF THE STATE OF PARA. **Report on the Vaccination Campaign against Foot-and-Mouth Disease.** November/2006 and January/February/2007 stages (Marajó), 2007.

AGUIAR, D.M., GENNARI, S.M., CAVALCANTE, G.T., LABRUNA, M.B., VASCONCELLOS, S.A., RODRIGUES, A.A.R., MORAES, Z.M., CAMARGO, L.M.A. Prevalence of anti-Leptospira *spp* antibodies in cattle in the municipality of Monte Negro, Western Amazonia. **Pesquisa Veterinària Brasileira, 26:**1-8, 2006.

AHMED, R. Leptospiras infection in lactating buffaloes. **Pakistan Veterinary Journal.** 10: 98, 1990.

ALEXANDER, A.D., EVANS, L.B., KEEN, B.C. Leptospira Butembo: a distinct leptospiral serotype. **Bacteriological Journal. 77:** 668-669, 1959.

ALMEIDA, L.P., MARTINS, L.F.S., BROD, C.S., GERMANO, P.M.L. Seroepidemiological survey of leptospirosis in environmental sanitation workers in an urban locality in southern Brazil. **Revista de Saùde Publica, 28**: 76-81, 1994.

ALVES, C.J., VASCONCELLOS, S.A., CAMARGO, C.R.A., MORAES, Z.M. influência de fatores ambientais sobre a proporção de caprinos sororreatores para leptosspirose em cinco centros de criaçao do estado da Paraiba, Brasil. **Archives of the Biological Institute. 63:** 11-18, 1996.

ARAÙJO, V.E.M., MOREIRA, E.C., NAVEDA, L.A.B., SILVA, J.A., CONTRERAS, R.L. Frequency of *anti-Leptospira interrogans* agglutinins in blood sera of cattle in Minas Gerais, from 1980 to 2002. **Arquivo Brasileiro de Medicina Veterinària e Zootecnia. 57:** 1-7, 2005.

BEER, J. Leptospirosis. **In**: **Infectious Diseases in Domestic Animals**. Vol. 2 Editora Roca, Sao Paulo, SP, p. 305-313, 1988.

BENNETT, R.M. A survey of dairy farmers' decisions concerning the control of leptospirosis. **The Veterinary Record, 129**: 118, 1991.

BENNETT, R.M. Decision supports models of leptospirosis in dairy herds**. The Veterinary Record, 132**: 59-61, 1993.

BIELANSK, A., SURUJBALLI, O, GOLSTEYN THOMAS, E., TANAKA. E. Sanitary status of oocytes and embryos collected from heifers experimentally exposed to Leptospira borgpetersenii serovar hardjobovis. **Animal Reproduction Science, 54**: 65-73, 1998.

BLAZIUS, R.D., ROMAO, P.R., BLAZIUS, E.M., SILVA, O.S. Occurrence of Leptospira spp. Soropositive stray dogs in Itapema, Santa Catarina. **Cadernos de Saùblica. 21:** 1952-1956, 2005.

BLOOD, D.C., HENDERSON, J.A., RADOSTITS, O.M. Diseases caused by *Leptospira spp.* **In: Clinica Veterinària**, 7ª ed. Rio de Janeiro, Guanabara Koogan, p.637646, 1991.

BOLIN, C.A., ZUERNER, R.L., TRUEBA, G. Comparison of three techniques to detect *Leptospira interrogans* serovar hardjo type *hardjobovis* in bovine urine. **American Journal of Veterinary Research, 50**: 1001-1003, 1989.

BOLIN, C.A., CASSELLS, J.A., ZUERNER, R.L., TRUEBA, G. Effect of vaccination with a monovalent *Leptospira interrogans* serovar hardjo type *hardjobovis* vaccine on type *hardjobovis* infection of cattle. **American Journal of Veterinary Research, 52**: 16391643, 1991.

BREM, S., KOPP, H., MEYER, P. Leptospira antibody detection in dog serum in the years 1985 to 1988. **Berl. Munch. Tierarztl. Wochenschr.** V. 103, n. 3: 115-120, 1990.

BROD, C.S., MARTINS, L.F.S., NUSSBAUM, A.A. Bovine leptospirosis in the southern region of the state of Rio Grande do Sul. **A Hora Veterinària. 84:** 15-20, 1995.

BROWN, P.D., GRAVECAMP, C., CARRINGTON, D.G., VAN DE CAMP, H., HARTSKEERL, R.A., EDWARDS, C.N., EVERARD, C.O., TERPSTRA, W.J., LEVETT, P.N. Evaluation of the polymerase chain reaction for early diagnosis of leptospirosis. **Journal Medical Microbilogy. 43:** 110-114, 1995.

CABALLERO, A.S, ROMERO, J.G, MÉNDEZ, E.G., TORRES, A.M. Estudio serológico para la deteccion de anticuerpos contra leptospiras en granado bovino lechero en los municipios de Coacalco, Teoloyucan, Zumpango, Melchor Ocampo y Cuautitlan, en el estado de México. **Revista Latinoamericana de Microbiologia. 31:**191-194, 1989.

CABRAL, K.G., LANGONI, H. *Leptospira spp.* in milk from normal and mastitic cows. **Napgama. Year III, 4:** 3-5, 2000.

CALDAS, E.M., SAMPAIO, M.B., TICHCENKO, L.M., CUNHA, J.B., CAMARA, J.Q., SANTOS, M.L. Anti-leptospira agglutinins in animal serum. **Archives of the School of Veterinary Medicine - UFBA. 2:** 83-98, 1977.

CALDAS, E.M., VIEGAS, S.A.R., SILVA, E.D., VASCONCELLOS, S.A., REIS, R.S. Comparative study between the macroagglutination test and microscopic serum agglutination, using

L. interrogans and *L. biflexa* antigens in the rapid diagnosis of leptospirosis in animals. **Arquivos da Escola de Medicina Veterinària - UFBA. 19:**155-176, 1997. CASCELLI, E.S., FABRIS, M., MARTINEZ, E.S., SARAVI, M.A., CACHIONE, R.A. An outbreak of leptospirosis in calves in the province of Buenos Aires and its vaccination control. **Revista Medicina Veterinaria de Buenos Aires, 60**: 258-262, 1979.

CHAUDHRY, J.I., KHAN, M.A., AKHTAR, T., KHAN, A.G., CHAUDHRY, M.S. Seroprevalence of leptospirosis in buffaloes. **Buffalo Journal, 1**: 65-71, 1996.

CICERONI, L., DANIELLO, P., RUSSO, N., PICARELLA, D., NESE, D., LAURIA, F., PINTO, A., CACCIAPUOTI, B. Prevalence of leptospire infections in buffalo herds in Italy.**The Veterinary Record. 137:** 192-193, 1995.

COCKRILL, W.R. Present and future of buffalo production in the world. **Buffalo Journal, 2**: 3-11, 1994.

CORRÊA, M.O.A. Human leptospirosis in Brazil. **International Journal of Zoonoses, 2:** 01-09, 1975.

CORRÊA, W.M. & CORRÊA, C.N. Leptospiroses, **In: Enfermidades Infecciosas dos Mamiferos domésticos,** 2 Ediçao, Editora Mèdica e Cientifica Ltda, Rio de Janeiro-RJ, p. 219-227, 1992.

CORTEZ, A., CASTRO, A.M.G., HEINEMANN, M.B., SOARES, R.M., LEITE, R.C., SCARCELLI, E., GENOVEZ, M.E., ALFFIERI, A.A., RICHTZENHAIN, L.J. Detection of nucleic acids *from Brucella spp. Leptospira spp.* bovine herpesvirus and bovine viral diarrhea virus, in aborted bovine fetuses and perinatal dead animals. **Arquivo Brasileiro de Medicina Veterinària e Zootecnia. 58:** 01-08, 2006.

CUNHA, E.L.P. Survey of *Leptospira spp.* in cattle and rodents on dairy farms and study of animal and human infection by serological analysis using the microscopic serum agglutination test. **Master's dissertation abstract.** Botucatu, Sao Paulo, Universidade Estadual Paulista, 2001, 75 p.

DEACON, N.J., LAH, M. The potential of the polymerase chain reaction in veterinary research and diagnosis. **Austrlian Veterinary Journal. 66:** 442-444, 1999.

DHALIWAL, G.S., MURRAY, R.D., DOBSON, H. Presence of antigen and antibodies in serum and genital discharges of cows from dairy herds naturally infected with *Leptospira interrogans* serovar *hardjo*. **Research in Veterinary Science. 60** (2): 163-167, 1996.

DIKKEN, H., KMETY, E. Serological typing methods of leptospires. **In: Methods in Microbiology. V. 11,** Academic Press. New York. Bergan Publishing House, p. 259-307, 1978.

DÓRIA, J.D., OLIVEIRA, N.L.H., CATHALA, E.E., FILHO, M.P. Serological studies on leptospirosis in cattle in the State of Bahia. **EPABA. 30:** 01-06, 1979.

DÓRIA, J.D., VIEGAS, S.A.S.A., VIEGAS, E.A., SANTOS, N.M., VIRGENS, N.C. Serological study of leptospirosis in cattle in the state of Bahia. **Archives of the Bahia School of Veterinary Medicine. 5:** 123-158, 1980.

ELLIS, W.A., O'BRIEN, J.J., NEILL, S.D., HANNA, J. Bovine leptospirosis: Serological findings in aborting cows. **The Veterinary Record, 110**: 178-180, 1982.

ELLIS, W.A. Bovine leptospirosis in the tropics: prevalence, pathogenesis and control.

Preventive Veterinary Medicine, 2: 411-421, 1984.

ELLIS, W.A., O'BRIEN, J.J., CASSELLS, J.A., NEILL, S.D., HANNA, J. Excretion of *Leptospira interrogans* serovar *hardjo* following calving or abortion. **Research in Veterinary Science, 39**: 296-298, 1985.

ELLIS, W.A., CASSELLS, J.A., DOYLE, J. Genital leptospirosis in bulls. **The Veterinary Record, 118**: 333, 1986.

ELLIS, W.A. & THIERMANN, A.B. Isolation of leptospires from the genital tracts of Iowa cows. **American Journal of Veterinary Research, 47**: 1694-1696, 1986.

ELLIS, W.A. & McDOWELL, S. Leptospirosis. In: **Pollution in Livestock Production Systems,** Wallingford, UK. ed. Dewi, I.A.; Axford, R.F.E.; Marai, I.F.M.; Omed, H. p 167-186, 1993.

ELLIS, W.A. Leptospirosis as a cause of reproductive failure. **In: Veterinary clinics of North America: Food animal practice.** USA. v.10, no.3, p.463-478, 1994.

ELLIS, W.A. International Committee on Systematic Bacteriology Subcommittee on the Taxonomy of *Leptospira.* **International Journal of Systematic Bacteriology, 45**: 872874, 1995.

FAINE, S. Leptospirosis in farm and domestic animals. In: **Guidelines for the control of leptospirosis,** Geneva: World Health Organization, p.54-57, 1982.

FAVERO, A.C.M., PINHEIRO, S.R., VASCONCELLOS, S.A., MORAIS, Z.M., FERREIRA, F., FERREIRA NETO, J.S. Serovars of leptospires prevalent in serological examinations of buffalo sheep, goats, horses, pigs and dogs from several Brazilian states. **Ciência Rural, 32**: 1-11, 2002.

FERESU, S.B., KORVER, H., RIQUELME, N., BARANTON, G., BOLIN, C.A. Two new leptospiral serovars in the Hebdomadis serogroup isolated from Zimbabwe cattle. **International Journal of Systematic Bacteriology. 46:** 694-698, 1996.

FREITAS, J.C., SILVA, F.G., OLIVEIRA, R.C., DELBEM, A.B., MULLER, E.E., ALVES, L.A., SERGIO, P. Isolation of *Leptospira spp* from dogs, bovine and swine naturally infected. **Ciência**

Rural. 34: 01-06, 2004.

FUNASA - FUNDAÇAO NACIONAL DE SAÙDE (Online). Available at http://www.funasa.gov.br. Accessed on 10/11/2003.

GALLEGO, M.I. & GALLEGO, J.F. Bovine leptospirosis. Serological diagnosis and control. **Revista Del CEISA, 1**: 49-68, 1994.

GANGLEAZZI, U.A., GARCIA, F.T., BLISKA, F.M.M., CIPOLLI, K.M.V., ARIMA, H.K. Production and consumption of buffalo meat in Brazil. **Revista da Carne. 314:** 01-14, 2003.

GARCIA, J.L., NAVARRO, I.T. Serologic evaluation of leptospirosis and brucellosis in patients living in the rural area of the municipality of Guaraci, Paranà, Brazil. **Revista da Sociedade Brasileira Medicina Tropical, 34**: 1-3, 2001.

GENOVEZ, M.E. Important considerations about *Leptospira Hardjo*. **Fort Dodge Newsletter - Cattle** - August, 1999.

GENOVEZ, M.E., OLIVEIRA, J.C., CASTRO, V., FERRARI, C.I.L., SCARCELLI, E., CARDOSO, M.V., PAULIN, L.M. GREGORY, L., LANÇA NETO, P. Increase in calving rate of nelore herds with endemic leptospirosis by progressive culling and vaccination. **Revista Brasileira de Reproduçâo Animal, 27**: 539-541, 2003.

GILES, N., HATHAWAY, S.C., STEVENS, A.E. Isolation of *Leptospira interrogans* serovar *hardjo* from a viable premature calf. **The Veterinary Record. 113**: 174-176, 1983.

GIORGI, W., TERUYA, J.M., SILVA, A.S., GENOVEZ, M.E. Leptospirosis: Results of serum agglutinations carried out at the Biological Institute of São Paulo, during the years 1974-1980. **O Biológico. 47**: 299-309, 1981.

GIRIO, R.J.S. Comparative study of four apathogenic leptospira strains used in a screening test for the serological diagnosis of *leptospirosis* in buffaloes (*Bubalus bubalis*). **Master's dissertation.** Sao Paulo, ICB - USP, 1984.

GIRIO, R.J.S., MATHIAS, L.A. Occurrence of leptospirosis in cattle herds producing type B milk in the northern region of the state of Sao Paulo. **Ciência Veterinària de Jaboticabal. 3**: 03-05, 1989.

GIRIO, R.J.S., SILVA, R.A.P., FRANCESCHINI, P.H., SCHALCH, U.M., SCHALCH, F.J. Study of the possible influence of leptospirosis on certain reproductive characteristics in dairy calves. **Ciência Veterinària de Jaboticabal. 4** (1): 0708, 1990.

GIRIO, R.J.S., PEREIRA, F.L.G., FILHO, M.M., MATHIAS, L.A., HERREIRA, R.C.P., ALESSI, A.C., GIRIO, T.M.S. Research into antibodies against Leptospira spp. in wild and feral animals in the Nhecolândia region, Mato Grosso do Sul, Brazil. Use of the immunohistochemical technique to detect the agent. **Ciência Rural. 34** (1): 01-08, 2004.

GRÉGORIE, N., HIGGINS, R., ROBINSON, Y. Isolation of leptospires from nephritic kidneys of beef cattle at slaughter. **American Journal of Veterinary Research. 48:** 370371, 1987.

HEINEMANN, M.B., GARCIA, J.F., NUNES, C.M., GREGORI, F., HIGA, Z.M.M., VASCONCELLOS, S.A., RICHTZENHAIN, L.J. Detection and differentiation of *Leptospira spp.* Serovars in bovine semen by polymerase chain reaction and restriction fragment length polymorphism. **Veterinary Microbiology, 73**: 261-267, 2000.

HOMEM, V.S.F. Brucellosis, leptospirosis and tuberculosis in Uruarà, PA, a municipality in the Eastern Amazon. A study of the bovine and human populations. **Master's dissertation,** Sao Paulo, SP, USP School of Veterinary Medicine and Zootechny, 1999, 74 p.

IBGE - BRAZILIAN INSTITUTE OF GEOGRAPHY AND STATISTICS. Agricultural Census - Municipal Livestock Survey - (Online). Available at http://www.sidra.ibge.gov.br/bda/pecua. Accessed on 10/11/2005.

JAWETZ, E., MELNICK, J.L., ADELBERG, E.A., BROONKS, G.F., BUTEL, J.S., ORNSTON, L.N. Spirochetes and other spiral microorganisms. In: **Medical Microbiology**, 18th Edition, Ed. Guanabara Koogan, Rio de Janeiro, RJ. p. 230-236, 1991.

JONES, D.D., BEJ, A.K. Detection of foodborne microbial pathogens using polymerase chain reaction methods. **In: Griffin & Griffin, PCR technology current innovation.** ed. Boca Raton, CRC, Press, p. 341-365, 1994.

JULIANO, R.S., CHAVES, N.S.T., SANTOS, C.A., RAMOS, L., SANTOS, H.Q., MEIRELES, L.R., GOTTSCHALK, S., CORREA FILHO, R.A. Prevalence and epidemiological aspects of bovine leptospirosis in dairy herds in the micro-region of Goiânia - GO. **Ciência Rural. 30:** 01-09, 2000.

KINGSCOTE, B.F. Leptospirosis in Livestock. **Canadian Veterinary Journal, 26**: 235236, 1985.

KHAN, M.A., KHAN, M.S. Seroprevalence of Leptospira interrogans in the aborting dairy buffaloes. **In: PROCEEDING OF WORLD BUFFALO CONGRESS** - india. 2: 57-60, 1988.

KOPCHA, M. & BARTLETT, P.C. Important zoonoses from direct contact with livestock. **Veterinary Medicine**, 370-374, 1997.

KORVER, H. Microscopic agglutination test (MAT) for the diagnosis of leptospirosis and serotyping of leptospiras. Available at http://www.vet.bg.ac.yu/lepto/lab/mat.html. Accessed on 13/09/2000.

LANGONI, H., MARINHO, M., BALDINI, S., SILVA, A.V., CABRAL, K.G., SILVA, E.R. Research of antileptospiral agglutinins in sheep sera in the State of Sao Paulo, Brazil, using macroagglutination plate tests and microscopic serum agglutination. **Revista Brasileira de Medicina Veterinària, 17**: 264-268, 1995.

LANGONI, H. DEL FAVA, C., ABRAL, K.G., SILVA, A.V., CHAGAS, S.A. Epidemiological survey on anti-leptospire agglutinins in buffaloes from Vale do Ribeira, SP, state (Brazil). **In: Proceeding of World Buffalo Congress,** 5 Caserta, Italy, p. 622625, 1997.

LANGONI, H., SOUZA, L.C., SILVA, A.V., LUVIZOTTO, M.C., PAES,[a] C., LUCHEIS, S.B. Incidence of leptospiral abortion in Brazilian dairy cattle. **Preventive Veterinary Medicine, 40**: 271-275, 1999.

LANGONI, H., MEIRELES, L.R., GOTTSCHALK, S. CABRAL, K.G., SILVA, A.V. Serological profile of bovine leptospirosis in regions of the state of Sao Paulo. **Archives of the Biological Institute (online).** Available at http//www.biologico.br. Accessed on 13/09/2000.

LEONARD, F.C., QUINN, P.J., ELLIS, W.A., O'FARREL, K. Duration of urinary excretion of leptospires by cattle naturally or experimentally infected with *Leptospira interrogans* serovar *hardjo*. **The Veterinary Record, 131**: 435-439, 1992.

LILENBAUM, W., SANTOS, M.R.C., BARBOSA, A.A.V. Leptospirosis in animal reproduction: II. Cattle in the state of Rio de Janeiro, Brazil. **Revista Brasileira Ciência Veterinària. 2** (1):1-6, 1995.

LINS, Z.C. Bacterial Diseases. **In: Infectious and Parasitic Diseases.** R. Veronesi (Ed.), 7th ed, Rio de Janeiro: Guanabara Koogan, p. 1146-1148, 1982.

LINS, Z.C., LOPES, M.L. Isolation of *Leptospira* from wild Forest animals in Amazonian Brazil. **In: Transactions of the Royal Society of Tropical Medicine and Hygiene, v. 78,** p. 124-126, 1984.

LINS, Z.C., LOPES, M.L., MAROJA, O.M. Epidemiology of leptospiroses with particular reference to the Brazilian Amazon. In: **Evandro Chagas Institute - 50 years. 1936 - 1986**, Belém-PA. p. 733-761, 1986.

LUCCHESI, P.M.A., ARROYO, G.H., ETCHEVERRIA, A.I., PARMA, A.E., SEIJO, A.C. Recommendations for the detection of Leptospira in urine by PCR. **Revista da Sociedade Brasileira de Medcina Tropical. 37:**01-05, 2004.

MACKINTOSH, C.G., SCHOLLUM, L.M., BLACKMORE, D.K., MARSHALL, R.B. Epidemiology of leptospirosis in dairy farm workers in the Manawatu. Part II. Acase- control study of high and low risk farms. **New Zealand Veterinary Journal. 30**: 73-76, 1982.

MADRUGA, C.R., AYCARDI, E., PUTT, N. Frequency of anti-leptospira agglutinins in beef cattle from the southern cerrado region of the state of Mato Grosso. **Arquivos da Escola de Veterinària da UFMG. 32:** 245-249, 1980.

MAGAJEVSKI, F.S., GIRIO, R.J.S., MATHIAS, L.A., MYASHIRO, S., GENOVEZ, M.E., SCARCELLI, E.P. Detection of *Leptospira spp.* in semen and urine of bulls serologically reactive to *Leptospira interrogans* serovar Hardjo. **Brazilian Journal of Microbiology. 36:** 01-08, 2005.

MARLER, R.J., COOK, J.E., KERR, A.I., KRUCKENBERG, S.M. Serologic survey for leptospirosis coyotes in northcentral Kansas. **Journal of the American Veterinary Medical Association. 175:** 906-908, 1979.

MARTiNEZ, G. B. Potentialities and threats by buffaloes on the Amazon floodplain. **1st Buffalo Symposium of Americas,** p 510-512, 2002.

McCLINTOCK, C.S., McGOWAN, M.R., CORNEY, B.G., COLLEY, J., SMYTHE, L., DOHNT, M., WOODROW, M. Isolation of *Leptospira interrogans* serovar hardjo and zanoni from a dairy herd in north Queensland. **Australian Veterinary Journal 70:** 393394, 1993.

MEDRONHO, R.A., CARVALHO, M.D., BLOCH, K.V., LUIZ, R.R., WERNWCK, G.L. **Epidemiologia.** Sao Paulo: Atheneu, 2002.

MÉRIEN, F., AMOURIAX, P.P., BARANTON, G., GIRONS, S. Polymerase chain reaction for detection of *Leptospira spp* in clinical samples. **Journal Clinical Microbiology, 30**: 2219-2224, 1992.

MÉRIEN, F., BARANTON, G., PEROLAT, P. Comparison of polymerase chain reaction with microagglutination test and culture for diagnosis of leptospirosis. **Journal Infection Disease. 172**: 281-285, 1995.

MILLER, D.A., WILSON, M.A., BERAN, G.W. Survey to estimate prevalence of *Leptospira interrogans* infection in mature cattle in the United States. **American journal of Veterinary research, 52**: 1761-1768, 1991.

MINEIRO, A.B.B. Anti-leptospira agglutinins in dairy cattle from the Parnaiba micro-region, Piaui. **Master's Degree Dissertation Summary.** Teresina - Piaui, Federal University of Piaui, 2003, 62p.

MINISTRY OF HEALTH. National Health Foundation. **Leptospirosis manual.** 2ª Edition, Brasilia, 98 p, 1995.

MIRAGLIA, F., MORAIS, Z.M., CORTEZ, A., MELVILLE, P.A., MARVULLO, V., RICHTZENHAIN, L.J., VISINTIN, J.A., VASCONCELLOS, S.A. Comparison of four antibiotics for inactivating leptospires in bull semen diluted in egg yolk extender and experimentally inoculated with *Leptospira santarosai* serovar guaricura. **Brazilian Journal of Microbiology. 34:** 01-09, 2003.

MOCH, R.W., EBNER, E.E., BARSOUM, L.S., BOTROS, B.A. Leptospirosis in Ethiopia: a serological survey in domestic and wild animals. **The Journal of Tropical Medicine and Hygiene. 78:** 38-42, 1975.

MOLNAR, E., SOUZA, H.E.M., MOLNAR, L. Leptospirosis in a buffalo herd in Amazonia. **XI BRAZILIAN CONGRESS OF ANIMAL REPRODUCTION. Proceedings**, p. 460, belo Horizonte, MG, 1995.

MOLNAR, E., MOLNAR, L., NEGRÂO, A.M.G., ROCHA, M.C. Considerações sobre o diagnóstico da leptospirose no homem e algumas espécies animais. **Revista Paraense de Medicina, 14**: 35-41, 2000.

MORAIS, M.H.F. Isolation of leptospira Hardjo in a bovine herd with reproductive problems. **Master's dissertation abstract.** Belo Horizonte, Minas Gerais, Federal University of Minas Gerais, 1994, 55 p.

MOREIRA, T.M.S. Prevalence of antileptospiral agglutinins in blood sera from the states of Parà and Amazonas - Brazil. **Master's dissertation.** Belo Horizonte, Federal University of Minas Gerais, 1982, 43p.

MOREIRA, E.C. Evaluation of methods for eradicating leptospirosis in dairy cattle. **Doctoral thesis.** Belo Horizonte, UFMG Veterinary School, 1994, 110 p.

MOURA CARVALHO, L.O.D.; LOURENÇO-JÙNIOR, J.B.; TEIXEIRA-NETO, J.F.; COSTA, N.A.; BAENA, A.R.C. Buffalo milk and meat production systems on a small farm in amazon. **1st Buffalo Symposium of Americas,** p 83-93, 2002.

MYBURG, J.G., NELSON, F.R., MECH, R.E. Serological reactions to leptospira species in buffalo (*Syncerus caffer*) from the Kruger National Park. **Onderst Australian Journal Veterinarian Research. 57:** 281-282, 1990.

NEGRÂO, A.M.G. Diagnosis of bovine leptospirosis in some regions of the State of Parà, Brazil. **Master's dissertation.** Belém, Parà, Universidade Federal do Parà, 1999, 96 p.

NEGRÂO, A.M.G., DIAS, H.L.T., SILVA, J.V., COSTA, S.C. Occurrence and predominant serotypes of leptospirosis in cattle and buffaloes in the State of Parà. **In: XXVIII BRAZILIAN CONGRESS OF VETERINARY MEDICINE**, Abstracts, Salvador, Bahia, p. 2001.

NEGRÂO, A.M.G., DIAS, H.L.T., COSTA, S.C.; SILVA, E.B., SANTOS, W.R.R. Seroprevalence of the leptospirosis in herds buffaloes in the of Parà state, Brazil. 1° **Buffalo Symposium of Americas,** p 382-386, 2002.

NEGRÂO, A.M.G., DIAS, H.L.T., SILVA, J.V., COSTA, S.C. Leptospirosis in buffaloes: seroprevalence of *Leptospira interrogans* serotypes hardjo and butembo in herds in the State of Parà - Brazil. **Revista Brasileira de Reproduçâo Animal, 27**: 549-551, 2003.

OIE - OFFICE INTERNATIONAL DES EPIZOOTIES. Available at http://www.oie.int/esp/norms. Accessed on 31/10/2001.

OLIVEIRA, A.A.F., MOTA, R.A., PEREIRA, G.C., LANGONI, H., SOUZA, M.I., NAVEGANTES, W.A., SA , M.E.P. Seroprevalence of bovine leptospirosis in Garanhuns municipal district, Pernanbuco State, Brazil. **Journal of Veterinary Research, 68**: 275279, 2001.

OLIVEIRA, D.R., SEIXAS, V.N.C., CARDOSO, E.C., VIANA, R.B., ARAÙJO, C.V., PEREIRA, W.L.A. Influence of mineral supplementation on the carcass yield of buffalo in the State of Parà, Brazil. MATSUDA Top Bùfalo. Available at http://www.bufalo.com.br/trabalhos/Oliveira 2005 sal matsuda. Accessed on 31/10/2005.

OOTEMAN, M.C. Composition of the PCR chain reaction with the microscopic serum agglutination reaction (SAM) and immunoenzymatic assay (ELISA-IgM) for the diagnosis of human leptospiroses. **Master's dissertation abstract.** Belo Horizonte, Minas Gerais, Federal University of Minas Gerais, 2001, 75 p.

ORR, H.S. & LITTLE, W.A. Isolation of leptospira of the serotype *hardjo* from bovine kidneys. **Research in Veterinary Science. 27**: 343-346, 1979.

PARMA, A.E., SEIJO, A., LUCCHESI, P.M., DEODATO, B., SANZ, M.E. Differentiation of pathogenic and non-pathogenic leptospires by means of the polymerase chain reaction. **Revista do Instituto de Medicina Tropical de Sao Paulo. 39:** 01-09, 1997.

PASSOS, E.C., VASCONCELLOS, S.A., ITO, F.H., YASUDA, P.H.,JUNIOR, R.N. Isolation of leptospires from hamster kidney tissue experimentally infected with *Leptospira interrogans* serotype pomona. Use of the Pasteur pipette technique and serial dilutions in Flether's culture medium treated with 5-fluorouracil or neomycin sufate. **Revista da Faculdade de Medicina Veterinària e Zootecnia da USP. 25:** 221-235, 1988.

PEREIRA, H.S., BLUME, H., SOLANO, R.F., NASCIMENTO, C. Incidence of leptospirosis in buffaloes in Maranhao. **Revista Brasileira de Reproduçâo Animal. 23:** 418-420, 1999.

PIRES, L. Polymerase chain reaction. **FAPESP - SP (on line)**. Available at http://www.fapesp.br/genes. Accessed on 07/12/2002.

PRADO, J.A. Immunoenzymatic and molecular biology methods applied to the diagnosis and control of infectious animal diseases. **A Hora Veterinària. 18:** 65-70, 1999.

PREGNOLATTO, B.P. Evaluation of gene-specific tests for the diagnosis of human leptospirosis. **Master's Degree Dissertation Summary. Sao Paulo,** University of Sao Paulo, 2001, 120 p.

QUINLAN, J.F. & McNICHOLL, V.J. Agalactia and infertility due to *Leptospira interrogans* serovar *hardjo* infection in a vaccinated dairy herd. **Irish Veterinary Journal, 46**: 97-98, 1993.

RATNAM, S., EVERARD, C.O.R., ALEX. C. A pilot study on the prevalence of leptospirosis in Tamilnadu state. **Indian Veterinary Journal. 71:** 1059-1063, 1994.

RIBEIRO, S.C.A., MOREIRA, E.C., GOMES, A.G., VALE, C. *Leptospira interrogans* infection on a farm in Minas Gerais, Brazil. **Arquivo Brasileiro de Medicina Veterinària e Zootecnia. 40** (2): 137-144, 1988.

RODRIGUES, C.G., MULLER, E.E., FREITAS, J.C. Bovine leptospirosis: serology in the Ieiteira basin of the Londrina region, Paranà, Brazil. **Ciência Rural. 29:** 01-08, 1999.

ROMERO, E.C., BILLERBECK, A.E.C., LANDO, V.S., CAMARGO, E.D., SOUZA, C.C., YASUDA, P.H. Detection of leptospira DNA in patients with aseptic meningitis by PCR. **Journal of Clinical Microbiology. 15:** 1453-1455, 1998.

SANDOVAL, L.A., ARRUDA, N.M., TERUYA, J.M., GIORGI, W., AMARAL, L.B.S., MAZANTI, M.T., ARRUDA, N.M. Study of buffaloes: prevalence of brucellosis and leptospirosis in the state of Sao Paulo, Brazil. **Biological. 45:** 209-212, 1979.

SANTA ROSA, C.A. Laboratory diagnosis of leptospirosis. **Revista de Microbiologia. 1** (2): 97-109, 1970.

SANTA ROSA, C.A., CASTRO, A.F.P., SILVA, A.S., TERUYA, J.M. Nine years of leptospirosis at the Sao Paulo Biological Institute. **Journal of the Adolfo Lutz Institute. 29/30:** 19-27, 1970.

SANTANA, A.O.B., OBA, E., LANGONI, E., URIBE, L.F.V. Anti-leptospiral agglutinins in oestrus-repeating bovine females. **Revista Brasileira de Reproduçao Animal. 21** (2): 169-172, 1997.

SCARCELLI, E., PIATTI, R.M., GENOVEZ, M.E., CARDOSO, M.V., CASTRO, V., FEDULLO, J.D.L., SIMON, F. Detection of *Leptospira spp* by the polymerase chain reaction (PCR) technique in clinical samples from captive-bred capuchin monkeys *(Cebus apella)*. **Archives of the Biological Institute, 67**. Abstract 038, supplement, 2000.

SCARCELLI, E., PIATTI, R. M., FEDULLO, J. D. L.; SIMON, F.; CARDOSO, M. V.; CASTRO, V., MIYASHIRO, S.; GENOVEZ, M. E. *Leptospira* spp detection by polymerase chain reaction (PCR) in clinical samples of captive black-capped capuchin monkey (*Cebus apella*). **Brazilian Journal of Microbiology, 34:** 143-146, 2003.

SHIMABUKURO, F.H., DOMINGUES, P.F., LANGONI, H., SILVA, A.V., PINHEIRO, J.P., PAVOVANI, C.R. Investigation of leptospira-carrying pigs by microbial isolation and polymerase chain reaction in kidney samples from serologically positive and negative animals for leptospirosis. **Brazilian Journal of Veterinary Research and Animal Science. 40:** 01-15, 2003.

SILVA, J.A., OLIVEIRA, P.R., CAMRGOS, C.R.M., FERNANDES, A.A., SILVA, M.B.O., COLICCHIO, A.L., ANDEREGG, P.I. Frequency of brucellosis and leptospirosis in dairy herds in the municipality of Esmedaldas - MG. **XXIII BRAZILIAN CONGRESS OF VETERINARY MEDICINE.** Proceedings. Olinda - PE, p.241, 1994.

SILVA, E.D. Evaluation of the macroagglutination reaction with *Leptospira interrogans* serovars in the search for agglutins in sera from dogs with clinical suspicion of leptospirosis. **Master's dissertation abstract.** Rio de Janeiro - RJ, Federal Rural University of Rio de Janeiro, 1998, 52 p.

SKILBECK, N.W. & DAVIES, W.D. Restriction endonuclease analysis of Australian isolates of *Leptospira interrogans* serovar *hardjo.* **Australian Veterinary Journal. 66** (6): 183-184, 1988.

SMITH, C.R., KETTERER, P.J., McGOWAN M.R., CORNEY, B.G. A review of laboratory techniques and their use in the diagnosis of *Leptospira interrogans* serovar *hardjo* infection in cattle. **Australian Veterinary Journal, 71**: 290-294, 1994.

SOUTH, P.J. & STOENNER, H.G. The control of outbreaks of leptospirosis in beef cattle by simultaneous vaccination and treatment with dihydrostreptomycin. **In: Annual meeting, U.S. Animal Health Association, 78,** 1974.

TAYLOR, M.J., ELLIS, W.A., MONTGOMERY, J.M., YAN, K.T., McDOWELL, S.W.J., MACKIE, D.P. Magnetic immuno capture PCR assay (MIPA): detection of *Leptospira borgpetersenii* serovar Hardjo. **Veterinary Microbiology. 56:** 135-145, 1997. TELÒ, P., AUTORINO, G., AMADDEO, D., TAGLIABUE, S., FINAZZI, G., PACCIARINI, M.L. Genetic characterization of a new leptospira belonging to serogroup Sejroe isolated from buffalo in Central Italy. **In: II International Leptospirosis Society Congress,** Maryslille, Australia, p. 77, 1999.

THIERMANN, A.B. Experimental leptospiral infections in pregnant cattle with organisms of the Hebdomadis serogroup. **American Journal Veterinary Research, 43**: 780-784, 1982.

THIERMANN, A.B. Bovine leptospirosis: Bacteriologic versus serologic diagnosis of cows at slaughter. **American Journal of Veterinary Research, 44**: 2244-2245, 1983.

THIERMANN, A.B., GARRETT, L.A. Enzyme-linked immunosorbent assay for the detection of antibodies to *Leptospira interrogans* serovar Hardjo and Pomona in cattle. **American Journal of Veterinary Research. 44:** 884-887, 1983.

THIERMANN, A.B. Leptospirosis: Current developments and trends. **Journal of American Veterinary Medical Association, 184**: 722-725, 1984.

UNIVERSITY OF BELGRADE. **Leptospira Home Page (on line).** Available at http://www.vet.bg.ac.yu/lepto. Accessed on 13/09/2000.

UPADHYE, A.S., KRISHNAPPA, G., AHMED, S.N. Leptospiral antibodies in aborted beffaloes. **Indian Veteinary Journal. 58:** 1, 1981.

UPADHYE, A.S., RAJASEKHAR, M., AHMED,, S.N., KRISHNAPPA, G. Isolation of Leptospira andamana from an active case of jaundice in a Buffalo. **Indian Veteinary Journal. 60:** 319-320, 1983.

VAN EYS, G.J.M., GRAVECAMP, C., GUERRITSEN, M.J., QUINT, W., CORNELISSEN, M.T.E., SCHEGGET, J., TERPSTRA, W.J. Detection of leptospirosis in urine by polymerase chain reaction. **Journal of Clinical Microbiology, 27:** 2258-2262, 1989.

VAN EYS, G.J.M., GUERRITSEN, M.J., KORVER, Q.H., SCHOONE, G.J., KROON, C.C.M., TERPSTRA, W.J. Characterization of serovars of the genus *Leptospira* by DNA hybridization with hardjobovis and Icterohaemorrhagiae recombinant probes with special attenction to serogroup Sejroe. **Journal of Clinical Microbiology, 20:** 1042-1048, 1991. VASCONCELLOS, S.A. The role of reservoirs in the maintenance of leptospirosis in nature. **Comunidade Cientifica da Faculdade de Veterinaria e Zootecnia da USP, 11**: 17-24, 1987.

VASCONCELLOS, S.A., BARBARINI JÙNIOR, O., CORTEZ, A., PINHEIRO, S.R., FERREIRA, F., FAVERO, A.C.M., FERREIRA-NETO, J.S. Bovine leptospirosis. Levels of occurrence and predominant serotypes in herds in the states of Minas Gerais, São Paulo, Rio de Janeiro, Paranà, Rio Grande do Sul and Mato Grosso do Sul, from January to April 1996. **Archives of the Biological Institute, 64**: 7-15, 1997.

VASCONCELLOS, S.A., OLIVEIRA, J.C.F., MORAIS, Z.M., BARUSELI, P.S., AMARAL, R., PINHEIRO, S.R., FERREIRA, F., FERREIRA-NETO, J.S., SCHONBERG, A., HARTSKEERL, R.A. Isolation of *Leptospira santarosai,* serovar

guaricura from buffaloes *(Bubalus bubalis)* in vale do Ribeira, Sao Paulo, Brazil. **Brzilian Journal Microbiology, 32**: 1-6, 2001.

VERONESI, R. Leptospiroses. **In: Doenças Infecciosas e Parasitarias,** 8ª Ed, Rio de Janeiro, Ed. Guanabara Koogan, p. 565-579, 1991.

VIDIC, B., LALIC, M., ZORICA, S., GRGIC, Z. Seroprevalence of *Leptospira interrogans* serovar Hardjo in cows and isolation from urine. **Acta Veterinaria. 47:** 15-22, 1997.

VIEGAS, E.A., VIEGAS, S.A.S.A., CALDAS, E.M. Anti-leptospira agglutinins in goat and sheep serum in the State of Bahia. **Archives of the School of Veterinary Medicine - UFBA. 5:** 20-34, 1980.

WEBER, A., WEBER, G., KRAUSS, H. Evaluation of the slide agglutination test for detection of leptospiral antibodies in serum samples of slaughter pigs. **Zentralbl. Bakteriology Mikrobiologic Hyg. 257:** 498-500, 1984.

WHITE, F.H., SULZER, K.R., ENGEL, R.W. Isolations of *Leptospira interrogans* serovar hardjo, balcanica and pomona from cattle at slaughter. **American Journal of Veterinary Research. 43:** 1172-1173, 1982.

WIKIPÉDIA - The Free Encyclopedia (online). Available at http://pt.wikipedia.org/wiki. Accessed on 23/11/2006.

WOODWARD, M.J., SWALLOW, C., KITCHING, A., DALLEY, C., SAYERS, A.R. *Leptospira hardjo* serodiagnosis: a comparison of MAT, ELISA and Immunocomb. **The Veterinary Record, 141**: 603-604, 1997.

YASUDA, P.H., SAMARA, S.I., PINTO, A.A. Anti-leptospira agglutinins in buffaloes in the State of Sao Paulo, Brazil. **In: ENCONTRO DE PESQUISAS VETERINARIAN** Jaboticabal, Sao Paulo. Abstracts. p. 105-106, 1982.

YASUDA, P.H.; STEIGERWALT, A.G.; SULZER, K.R.; KAUFMANN, A.F.; ROGERS, F.; BRENNER, D.J. Deoxyribonucleic acid relatedness between Serogroups and serovars in the family *Leptospiraceae* with proposals for seven new *Leptospira* species. **International Journal of Systematic Bacteriology, 37**: 407-415, 1987.

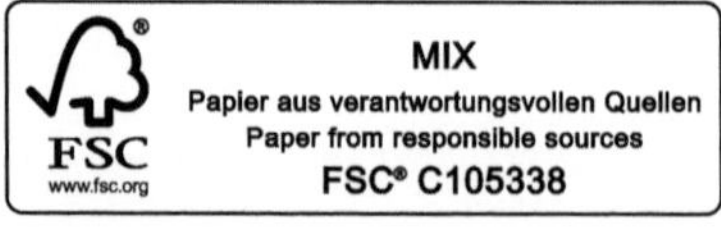

Printed by Books on Demand GmbH, Norderstedt / Germany